THE
ACID WATCHER
COOKBOOK

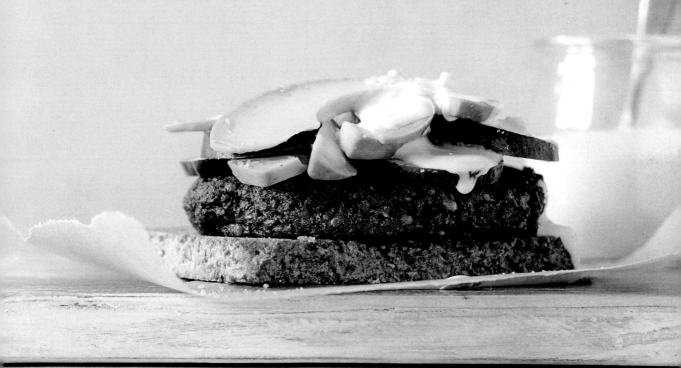

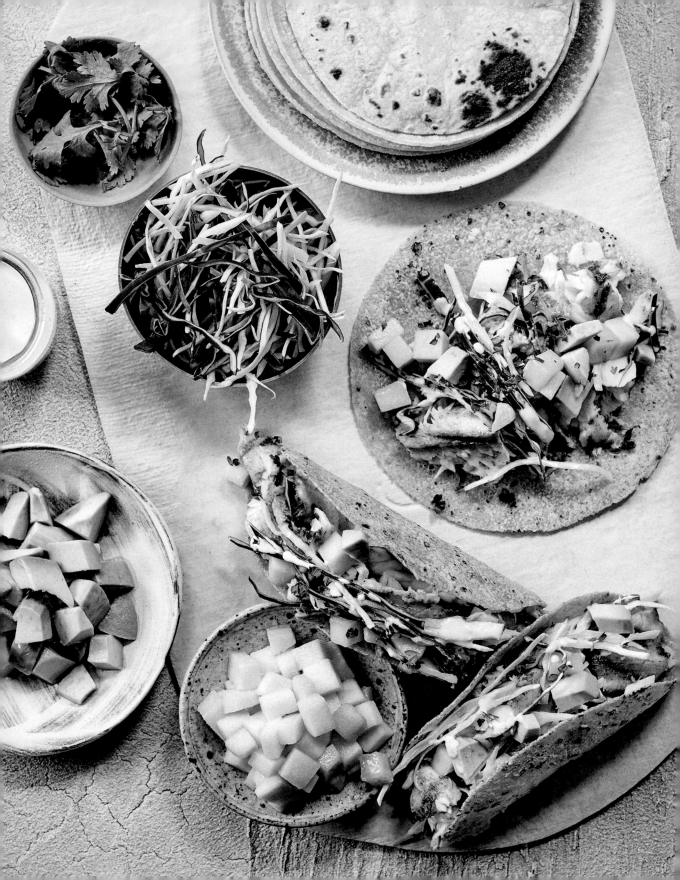

THE
ACID WATCHER
COOKBOOK

100+ DELICIOUS RECIPES
——— *to* **PREVENT** *and* **HEAL** ———
ACID REFLUX DISEASE

JONATHAN AVIV, MD
with SAMARA KAUFMANN AVIV, MA

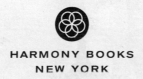

HARMONY BOOKS
NEW YORK

Published in the United States by Harmony Books, an imprint of Random House, a division of Penguin Random House LLC, New York.
harmonybooks.com

Harmony Books is a registered trademark, and the Circle colophon is a trademark of Penguin Random House LLC.

Library of Congress Cataloging-in-Publication Data is available upon request.

ISBN 978-0-525-57556-6
Ebook ISBN 978-0-525-57557-3

Printed in China

Book and cover design: SONIA PERSAD

Cover and interior photography: ROBERT BREDVAD

10 9 8 7 6 5 4 3 2 1

First Edition

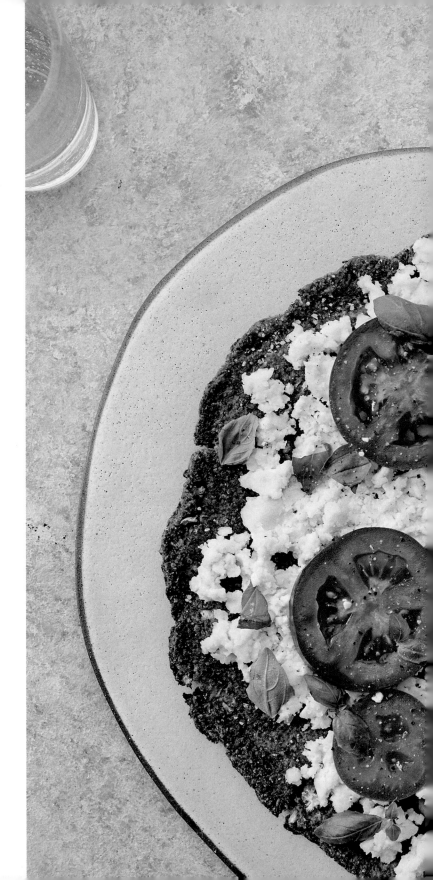

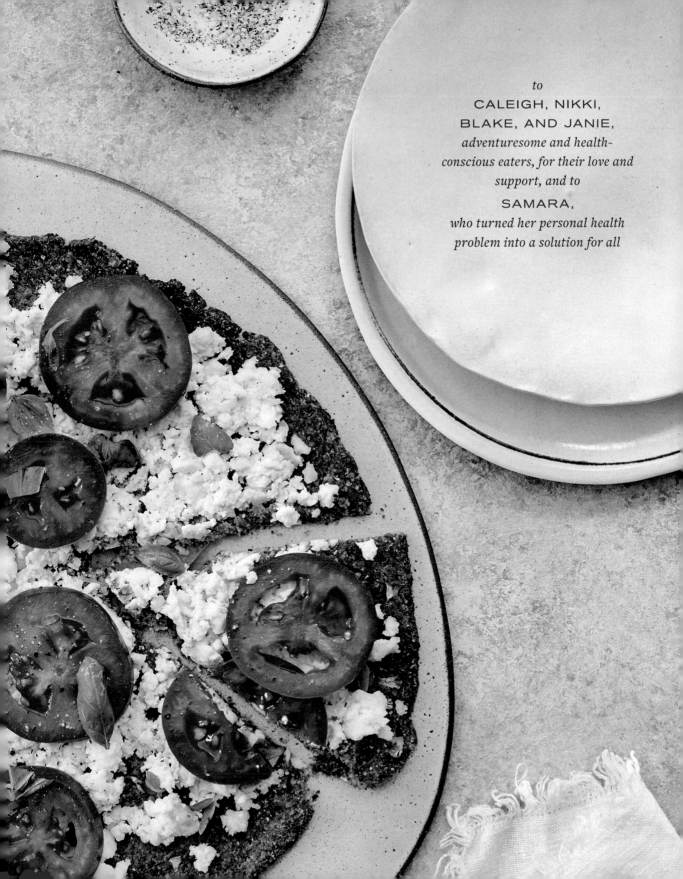

to
**CALEIGH, NIKKI,
BLAKE, AND JANIE,**
*adventuresome and health-
conscious eaters, for their love and
support, and to*
SAMARA,
*who turned her personal health
problem into a solution for all*

CONTENTS

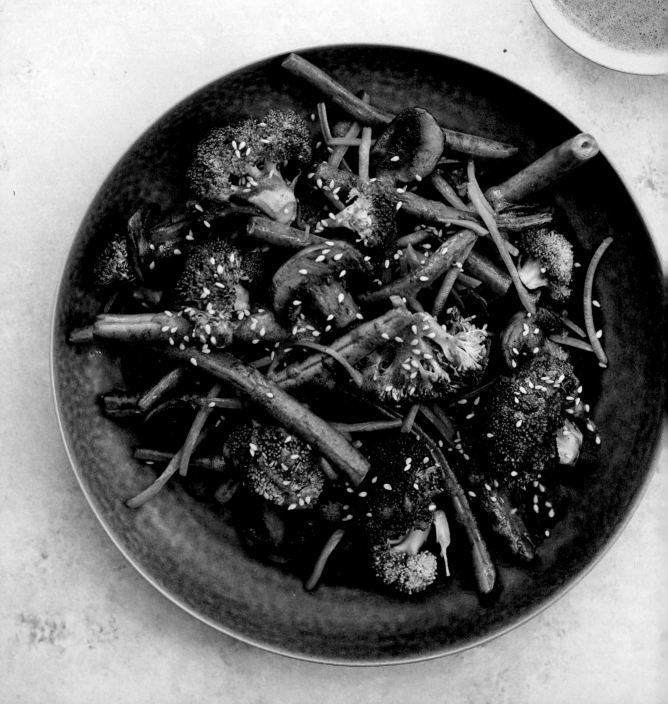

INTRODUCTION

WHY AN ACID WATCHER DIET COOKBOOK?

"Doctor Aviv, I can't stand my hoarse, raspy voice and constant throat clearing! I'm always coughing, and I have a constant lump in my throat. What can I do?"

As a practicing ear, nose, and throat physician specializing in voice and swallowing disorders, I have heard these laments from frustrated patients for many years. These symptoms are too often the result of acid reflux disease, a condition that affects over seventy-five million Americans and over a billion people worldwide. Acid reflux can present as heartburn or throat symptoms, with hoarseness, coughing, frequent throat clearing, and postnasal drip. Unfortunately, the solutions offered (a combination of medication and lifestyle changes) were unsatisfactory for my patients. It became apparent that the prolonged use of medications to reduce acid production by the stomach could lead to unacceptable side effects. I believed that the best and safest way to treat this disease was to come up with a food-based solution, which led to the creation of the Acid Watcher Diet.

In *The Acid Watcher Diet*, I introduced a twenty-eight-day low-acid, high-fiber, nutritionally balanced eating plan that helped heal the body from the damage of acid reflux disease by replacing acidic foods with alkaline foods.

As I was writing *The Acid Watcher Diet*, a new study came out showing that when an individual ingests an acidic substance, a *body-wide* inflammatory response takes place. This means that acid damage actually contributes to conditions *throughout the body* that are caused by chronic inflammation.

What was thought for years to be a limited response to acidic foods had to be reexamined. It was now apparent that we needed to create recipes that would neutralize acidic foods. *The Acid Watcher Diet* introduced this concept.

After *The Acid Watcher Diet* was published, I heard from followers of the diet all over the world, calling for more variety across the entire spectrum of foods. So the next step was to create a cookbook that would expand the diet's principles to include foods and flavors that were previously "forbidden," for instance, using tomato, citrus, and even vinegar in highly specific ways by combining (cooking, mixing, blending) them with alkaline foods so that their acidity is neutralized, without losing their flavor. I wanted to create tasty, healthy, anti-inflammatory recipes that have applications not only for acid reflux sufferers but also for anyone who loves to eat.

Another key step to creating a more appealing and effective anti-inflammatory diet was to offer dairy-free alternatives. Casein, found in cow's milk and cow's milk–based cheeses, is inflammatory and often particularly bothersome to those with acid reflux disease. In order to replace animal-based cheese with preservative-free, homemade plant-based "cheese" and "cheese sauces," I began working with Samara Kaufmann Aviv and experimenting with different types of nuts. To get that tangy cheese-like flavor, it became clear that we needed to add an acid. So began the trial and error of using different combinations of nuts with amounts of lemon, vinegar, and/or mustard until the robust, piquant flavor of cheese, with the appropriate mouthfeel, was attained. This formed the basis for many of the plant-based cheese substitutes found in this cookbook, such as "Mac 'n' Cheese" sauce (page 148) and "Caesar" salad dressing (page 129).

What ultimately resulted from this relentless series of food trials was Acid Watcher "pHriendly" food that widens the scope of variety and tastes, while keeping the acidity always above pH 4 (i.e., Maintenance Phase–compatible) and often above pH 5 (Healing Phase–safe).

The genesis of this nascent food science began several years ago with my coauthor's first sinus infection.

SAMARA'S STORY

For years, Samara had complained of sinus pressure in her face, postnasal drip with thick mucus trickling down into her throat, frequent throat clearing, and hoarseness with coughing. But it was the incessant throat clearing that drove Samara, and everyone around her, mad—at the movies, at the theater, at work, with friends, with family, on job interviews.

Each physician Samara sought counsel with advised different variations of multiple over-the-counter drugs, then prescription antihistamines, nasal steroid sprays, antihistamine sprays, allergy pills—though no allergies to foods or to the environment were ever found in formal testing. She underwent numerous courses of antibiotics.

A computed tomography (CT) scan of the sinuses early on in the duration of all these symptoms did indeed show some thickening of the normally paper-thin maxillary, or cheek, sinus lining. Samara's doctors felt that the abnormally thick sinus lining was the source of her troubling throat symptoms and diagnosed her with an awful case of postnasal drip due to allergies.

She underwent sinus surgery after eight years with the same symptoms, and post-op care lasted for months. She figured it would be worth it to be able to go to the movies without having to arm herself with an array of cough drops, throat sprays, nasal sprays, antihistamine pills, and the proverbial box of tissues. If that were only the case.

The throat symptoms in particular persisted.

Finally, a member of Samara's family said to her, "I think you have acid reflux. I would try the Acid Watcher Diet."

Samara thought the idea of a "stomach" condition causing her sinus and throat problems was absurd. She never once—ever—had heartburn, that searing feeling of what seems like a fireball irritating the chest, sometimes even a burning sensation going up into the throat.

Further, during the decade plus of addressing her "sinus" symptoms, no doctor had ever asked her what she was eating and drinking. No one ever questioned the nightly glass or two of wine with, or without, dinner or the spritz of lemon or lime that seemed to accompany every glass of water at every meal she ever enjoyed. There were no questions regarding the type of salad dressing used on the tomato and raw onion salad that was a staple of her diet, nor even a single inquiry about the bottled iced tea that quenched her thirst during her workday and occasionally during her workouts. No one asked about her habit of grabbing something to eat when finally arriving home after a long day, then lying down, exhausted, on her couch immediately afterward.

As it turns out, said family member was correct. He also had been suffering for ages with hoarseness, frequent throat clearing, excess throat mucus, and a lump sensation in the throat before visiting me for an exam. I placed an ultra-small camera, the size and softness of a shoelace, into his nose to examine his nose lining and throat. Lo and behold, it looked as if an IED had exploded in his throat.

I saw massive swelling everywhere: in the throat, in the vocal cords, and in the nose. In fact, the back of the throat was swollen with multiple small ridges of tissue, and it looked like a series of cobblestones. This type of acid-induced swelling is called, appropriately enough, "cobblestoning." It is not a death sentence and it is not permanent. In fact, with proper dietary control and lifestyle adjustments, the cobblestoning will disappear and the throat will return to its normal smooth structure. In addition to the throat ridges, there was swelling of the back of the vocal cord region, in a narrow area of the throat where the larynx (vocal cord organ) sits at the top of the esophagus. This swelling looked like the Michelin man or Jabba the Hut, with swollen rings of tissue heaped up on one another. These horizontal stripes of layered swollen tissue are called "tiger striping," which is also reversible. I advised him to follow the dietary and lifestyle changes of the Acid Watcher Diet. Symptoms began to improve. It must have made an impression.

Samara's throat was eventually examined and did indeed show multiple signs of inflammation: tiger striping, cobblestoning, swollen vocal cords, postnasal drip. She started the Acid Watcher Diet, and finally her throat symptoms began to resolve.

Fortuitously, Samara had spent her childhood years cooking with her late mother, who was a fantastic, adventuresome cook. In addition, Samara had a substantial background in the biological sciences. She was now able to combine her culinary skills with her science background, and, working together, we began to create recipes based on the Acid Watcher Diet principles that vastly expanded the original tenets of the diet.

For example, we noticed that traditional guacamole and hummus without onion or garlic did not bother us, so we began applying the principles of neutralization of acidic foods to these classic dishes. By gradually increasing the volumes of lime and lemon juice used in the traditional preparation of these dishes, we were able to achieve amounts of acid that allowed the dishes to retain their authenticity and flavor while keeping the pH well above 4.

The neutralization concepts were taken further with respect to acidic desserts that contain raspberry, for example. We found that this acidic ingredient could be "safely" used by cooking raspberries with different types of flours, which led to the creation of numerous Acid Watcher–compatible sweets and treats.

As a result of these initial rounds of "food experiments," we continued to create more and more recipes that ultimately formed the basis of this cookbook.

PREPARATION AND PRINCIPLES

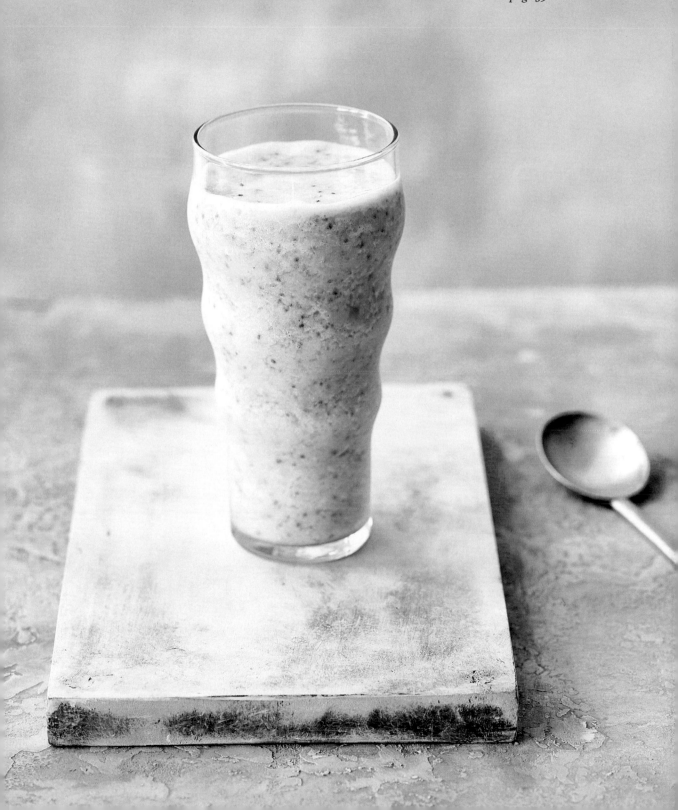

ORANGE CREAM SMOOTHIE,
page 39

WHAT IS THE ACID WATCHER DIET?

Many people believe that the one and only symptom of acid damage is heartburn. As we discovered in *The Acid Watcher Diet,* it's a misleading and often dangerous belief. As we saw with Samara's story, the "hidden" symptoms of acid damage can also include the following:

- hoarseness
- a chronic, nagging cough
- a sore throat that appears out of nowhere
- the feeling of a lump stuck in your throat
- postnasal drip
- allergies
- shortness of breath
- abdominal bloating

We know now that the problem is not just the acid that goes up the esophagus from your stomach, but the acid that comes down the esophagus when you ingest acidic and processed foods and beverages. Changing your diet can have life-changing effects, putting an end to the symptoms that are the result of years' worth of damage to your throat and esophagus.

The Acid Watcher Diet is a *low-acid, high-fiber,* nutritionally balanced diet that contains high-quality proteins, carbohydrates, and fat. It is not a deprivation diet. It will heal tissues damaged by dietary acid by eliminating high-acid processed foods from your diet and replacing them with natural low-acid alternatives. Another key feature of the Acid Watcher Diet is eating "on time." The kitchen closes at 7:30 p.m. That means that the diet's recommended five meals a day—three regular meals plus two mini meals—should be eaten over a twelve- to thirteen-hour time span. This is best accomplished from 6:30 a.m. to 7:30 p.m.

The Acid Watcher Diet is divided into two phases, a twenty-eight-day Healing Phase followed by the Maintenance Phase. During the Healing Phase, you'll enjoy foods with a pH of 5 and higher, including lean animal proteins, whole grains, and a range of fruits and vegetables. Foods that promote indigestion and acidification will be eliminated, including carbonated beverages, alcohol, caffeine, chocolate, mint, raw onion, and garlic. This way, you'll give your body time to recover from years of acid damage. With the three complete meals and two mini meals per day, you don't have to worry about feeling hungry or deprived.

For the Maintenance Phase, the goal is to eat foods above pH 4, and it can be extended for as long as you like so that you can take back your health for good. You'll be able to reintroduce caffeine, along with cooked garlic and onions, into your diet.

As you may already know, acidity and alkalinity are measured on the pH scale, which runs from 1 (extremely acidic) to 14 (extremely alkaline). Every substance below pH 7 is considered acidic, while everything above pH 7 is considered alkaline. Your body works hard to keep its pH at 7.4. Foods and drinks below pH 5, and especially below pH 4, activate a digestive enzyme called *pepsin*. Pepsin, normally located in the stomach, breaks down protein when exposed to acidity. The stomach has a pH of close to 2, which is very acidic, so pepsin is very active in the stomach.

However, pepsin can "float" out of the stomach and migrate to other areas of the body such as the esophagus, lungs, throat, vocal cords, nose, and sinuses. Consequently, when one consumes foods and beverages below pH 4, pepsin gets "turned on" and causes inflammation in those areas. During the Healing Phase, you'll heal acid injury with foods above pH 5, then maintain healing and prevent inflammation in the Maintenance Phase with foods above pH 4.

As with all diets, food plans, and holistic approaches to wellness, please discuss any possible changes in your diet and lifestyle with your doctor before embarking on your own.

We have updated the first four main principles of the Acid Watcher Diet here.

ACID WATCHER DIET PRINCIPLE #1: ELIMINATE ACID TRIGGERS

The first principle in the Healing Phase is to eliminate these "dirty dozen" food items:

1 **CARBONATED SODAS** These include the very acidic sugar and diet sodas, flavored club soda, and unflavored sparkling water. (In the Maintenance Phase, generally, unflavored sparkling water is okay. However, certain brands of sparkling waters, e.g., LaCroix, are below pH 4 and therefore should be avoided in the Maintenance Phase as well.)

2 **BOTTLED ICED TEA** Is full of acidified preservatives.

3 **CITRUS FRUITS** *No "non-neutralized" citrus* (lemon, lime, orange, grapefruit, pineapple) or other acidic fruits below a pH of 4, such as green apple, red and black berries (strawberry, raspberry, and blackberry), pomegranate, and cranberry.

Instead, use neutralization techniques, as you will see in the recipe section, so that citrus and acidic fruits can be used. Also, one may cook with citrus, as the cooking process burns off the acidity.

4 **TOMATO, TOMATO SAUCE, AND TOMATO PASTE** Although tomato has a large number of lycopenes, a natural antioxidant, it is acidic (pH 4 to 5). If you are concerned that giving up tomatoes means giving up a vital source of lycopene, don't worry; other sources of lycopene (such as watermelon) are allowed in the Healing Phase. In the Maintenance Phase, *raw tomatoes are allowed,* but tomato sauce and paste must still be avoided—except when used from the recipes in Section 2 (page 30).

5 **VINEGAR** *No vinegar is allowed,* including the notorious apple cider vinegar, raspberry wine vinegar, and red wine vinegar. Vinegar is extremely acidic because of the fermentation process it undergoes, and all varieties are pepsin activators. However, one may cook with vinegars, as the heating process in combination with other ingredients will typically mitigate vinegar's acidity. Also, as shown in some Healing Phase recipes, vinegar's acidity can be neutralized by the precise combination of additional ingredients.

6 **ALCOHOL** Alcohol, especially wine, is off-limits during the Healing Phase, because it is a carminative, meaning it loosens the lower esophageal sphincter (LES) muscle, thus allowing acidic stomach contents to "escape." And, in the case of wine, it is very acidic. Wine, measuring from pH 2.9 to pH 3.9, is not suitable for any phase of the Acid Watcher Diet. However, one may cook with wine.

Certain spirits are above pH 7, such as vodka and gin, so limited amounts are permitted in the Maintenance Phase. Tequila, because of the fermenting process, is often quite acidic and generally should be avoided in both phases of the Acid Watcher Diet.

7 **CAFFEINE** Coffee and caffeinated tea are off-limits during the Healing Phase, but also be aware of other products containing caffeine, such as over-the-counter and prescription medications, alcoholic beverages, and desserts. Wherever it is present, caffeine is an LES loosener and increases acid production by the stomach.

8   CHOCOLATE   This high nutritional-value indulgence is bad for Acid Watchers, especially those with heartburn. It contains methylxanthine, which loosens the LES and increases hydrochloric-acid production by the stomach. The good news is that the Acid Watcher Diet allows carob, a natural chocolate alternative that is just as delicious in homemade desserts.

   A note of caution with respect to caffeine and chocolate: While coffee and chocolate are not acidic (they are actually around pH 6), caffeine causes loosening of the lower esophageal muscle and increases acid production by the stomach. For the Maintenance Phase, a cup of coffee and a square of dark chocolate are permissible, as long as they don't make one symptomatic.

9   KETCHUP, MUSTARD, AND MAYO   Instead, use Acid Watcher–friendly substitutes such as Beet Ketchup (page 183), Creamy Dressing (page 164), and Caesar Dressing (page 129). Creating direct mustard substitutes has been challenging, as mustard is quite acidic and poorly tolerated by most individuals with acid reflux disease.

10   MINT   This is a powerful carminative, and the Acid Watcher Diet restriction applies to the herb itself, its variation as a spice, and flavored chewing gums and hard candies.

11   RAW ONION   This is another powerful carminative that loosens the LES, leaving the door open for refluxed acid. It is also a fructan, which means that it causes the intestines to absorb water, thereby causing bloating. During digestion, onion produces gassiness, especially if it is consumed raw. You should stay away from it completely during the Healing Phase. The good news is that onion that is cooked over high heat is reintroduced in the Maintenance Phase.

12   RAW GARLIC   Like raw onion, raw garlic is a carminative and a fructan and is therefore off-limits during the Healing Phase of the diet. The rules for onion apply to garlic as well, so in its cooked form, one can use it in the Maintenance Phase.

ACID WATCHER DIET PRINCIPLE #2:
REIN IN REFLUX-GENERATING HABITS

This means eliminate substances and practices that trigger acid reflux:

1   **ELIMINATE ALL SMOKING**   Cigarettes and other sources of inhaled smoke, including e-cigarettes, are carcinogens, LES looseners, and gastric acid release stimulants. You can't get rid of acid reflux or heal the damage to your esophageal tissue if you continue smoking.

2   **DROP PROCESSED FOOD**   Preservation methods in prepackaged, jarred, processed, and canned foods require the use of chemicals that are inherently acidic or have properties that loosen the LES. I allow three exceptions in the Acid Watcher Diet: canned tuna, chickpeas, and beans. Canned tuna must be water-packed and drained before using. Canned beans must be organic and thoroughly washed to eliminate traces of acidified liquids. The exception is aquafaba, the liquid in canned chickpeas (see the Real Hummus recipe, page 87).

In addition, *no processed or refined flours.* No white flour. No panko bread crumbs. Instead, use non-refined flours like almond (page 159), coconut, 100 percent whole-wheat flour, oat flour, organic quinoa flour, or organic corn flour.

3   **FORGET FRIED FOODS**   You probably already know that this method of cooking is not good for you because it adds bad fats and empty calories into your diet. What you may not know is that deep-frying oxidizes food, contributing to the proliferation of free radicals in your body, thereby setting the stage for chronic inflammation. Fried food is also a notorious LES loosener, which is why so many of us feel the regurgitation effect after eating it.

4   **EAT ON TIME**   An Acid Watcher should eat frequently but thoughtfully. During both the Healing Phase and the Maintenance Phase, you should eat three meals and two mini meals per day between 6:30 a.m. and 7:30 p.m. Although the Acid Watcher Diet is not portion controlled, you should not overeat because a stomach that is too full is a source of increased intra-abdominal pressure that can force open the LES. Close the kitchen at 7:30 p.m. to give your stomach three to four hours to digest food before you lie down.

ACID WATCHER DIET PRINCIPLE #3: PRACTICE THE RULE OF 5

The Rule of 5 means that for the Healing Phase, you should consume foods with a pH value of 5 and higher. This eliminates most canned and jarred products, as the preservatives and chemicals used to increase shelf life dramatically lower the pH value of any food. Scientific evidence has shown that most substances registering below 5 on the pH scale—and particularly those that dip below 4—are the most powerful activators of pepsin. However, the Rule of 5 is more inclusive than it is exclusive. You'll see a broad range of foods in the following list, and it includes plenty of lean proteins, whole grains, fruits and vegetables, condiments, and spices. Because the Acid Watcher Diet is about balance and moderation as opposed to deprivation, it doesn't exclude carbs, healthy fat, or protein. The only target for removal is highly acidic and processed food.

Here is a sampling of foods that measure pH 5 or higher:

FISH   salmon, halibut, tilapia, trout, flounder, branzino, sole

POULTRY   chicken breast, ground turkey, eggs

VEGETABLES AND HERBS   spinach, romaine lettuce, arugula, curly kale, bok choy, broccoli, asparagus, celery, cucumbers, zucchini, eggplant, yellow squash, potato, sweet potato, carrots, beets (fresh or pre-cooked), mushrooms, basil, cilantro, parsley, rosemary, thyme, sage

RAW FRUIT   banana, Bosc and Asian pear, papaya, cantaloupe, honeydew, watermelon, lychee, avocado

DRIED FRUIT   dates, Turkish apricots, shredded coconut

NUTS AND SEEDS   cashews, pecans, pistachios, walnuts, pumpkin seeds, sesame seeds, almonds, pine nuts

SPREADS   fresh, raw, organic peanut butter and almond butter

CHEESE   Parmesan and hard cheeses are permitted in small amounts. In general we would like to minimize cow's milk–derived products, including yogurt, as they tend to be inflammatory due to the casein protein they contain. If one desires yogurt, consider coconut milk–based yogurt brands such as Anita's and Coyo.

BREAD AND GRAINS   old-fashioned rolled oats, whole-grain pasta, 100 percent whole-grain bread, whole-grain wheat flour

SWEETENERS   No refined sugar or artificial sweeteners, including coconut sugar, stevia, or agave. The Acid Watcher Diet is a low-sugar diet. If you use sweeteners, use them sparingly. Limit yourself to either manuka honey or 100 percent pure organic maple syrup. To sweeten certain dishes, we prefer using whole foods such as dates, bananas, and dried apricots.

CONDIMENTS   Celtic salt, tamari, citrus zest, pure vanilla extract, white miso paste. These are options that provide endless variations for satisfying meals. No added oils besides cold-pressed extra-virgin olive oil and the occasional coconut oil are allowed. Instead, use natural oils from whole foods as much as possible. For instance, chicken tenders "breaded" in hempseed and almond flour (page 159) bake beautifully sans oil. Organic unsalted butter can be used sparingly in certain specific recipes.

ACID WATCHER DIET PRINCIPLE #4: MAKE POSITIVE FOOD CHOICES

The Acid Watcher Diet is popular with patients who are not fond of rigid portion control and calorie counting, and I am one of them. Don't get me wrong; I am not advocating consuming huge meals. Meals and snacks should be sensible in size, and you will find that over time you will want to eat less because you will be consuming more fiber and spacing your meals in reasonable intervals to prevent hunger from setting in. Remember that the Acid Watcher Diet provides you with all the macronutrients that your body needs, and when you eat a macronutrient-inclusive diet, you ensure greater appetite satisfaction. You also get to experience other positive side effects, such as diminished bloating, a trimmer belly, and more energy. To obtain quick results:

1 **Introduce more fiber into your diet.** Fiber is crucial, as it performs the function of a broom that sweeps all the waste from your stomach and intestines, aiding in healthy digestion and esophageal protection. By increasing your fiber consumption, you can leave the food cravings—and extra pounds—behind. You don't need to rely on supplements to increase your fiber intake.

2 **Eat a daily minimum of 1 pound of vegetables above pH 5, half of which should be consumed raw.** One pound may seem like a lot, but if you enjoy these vegetables throughout the day, you'll find it's easily doable. For example, five medium carrots weigh approximately 1 pound; consume half of these raw as snacks, and include the rest in a soup or stir-fry later in the day.

3 **Eat a daily minimum of ½ pound of raw fruit above pH 5.**

4 **Be aware of borderline pH-value foods that are bad for Acid Watchers.** Reflux-inducing substances may include condiments and natural products that are pH friendly (pH 5 and higher) but should be avoided by people with acid reflux. Among these are items listed in Principle #1: coffee, onions, tomato sauce, citrus fruit, vinegar, garlic, mint, and chocolate. But if you have acid reflux, you must also beware of the following items:

BERRIES   Red (strawberries, raspberries) and black (blackberries) berries are below pH 4, so they should be avoided in both phases of the diet. Berries are, however, allowed in both phases *if* they are balanced by acid neutralizers such as almond milk, non-GMO (non-genetically modified organism) soy milk, rice milk, and coconut milk. Notably, blueberries, which are generally above pH 4, are permitted in the Maintenance Phase.

HONEY   Its pH value is slightly below 5, so it is not allowed in the Healing Phase unless it is combined with acid neutralizers such as nut butters or raw animal protein (as in a marinade).

SPICES   Spices such as chili spice, chili powder, ground chiles, red pepper flakes, or jalapeño contain a chemical called capsaicin that is particularly inflammatory and can temporarily paralyze stomach movement. Instead, use spices such as cumin, paprika, coriander, turmeric, ground cloves, cinnamon, and ground ginger, as they are all fine during the Maintenance Phase.

PEPPERS   These are carminatives (looseners of the LES) so should be avoided in the Healing Phase. I do allow the introduction of cooked or raw bell peppers in the Maintenance Phase.

SEED OILS   *Canola, safflower, sesame,* and *sunflower* oils are inflammatory because their heat-based extraction process involves the use of chemicals and preservatives. I recommend cold-pressed extra-virgin olive oil or coconut oil.

5   **Balance your daily vegetable and protein intake.** Practicing positive food choices means placing greater emphasis on vegetable intake. If you eat poultry or fish for lunch, you should consume a vegetarian dinner. Conversely, a vegetarian lunch may be followed by a poultry or fish dinner. The rationale for eating at least one vegetarian meal a day is that higher consumption of vegetables (as well as fruit) is associated with a lower risk of mortality, particularly cardiovascular mortality. It is also another way to maximize your fiber intake.

6   **Substitute products wisely.**

- Choose grass-fed and/or organic over farmed animal protein.
- Choose a higher omega-3 to omega-6 ratio in seafood with the easiest rule of thumb being to consume *wild* seafood as compared to *farmed* seafood.
- Choose organic fruits and vegetables unless they have thick protective skin.
- Choose organic peanut butter, preferably freshly ground, as processed, industrially made peanut butter is more acidic.

- Replace processed table salt, which has been depleted of its essential minerals, with Celtic salt. In contrast to highly processed table salt whose crystals undergo an extreme chemical transformation in which they lose nearly all of their nutrients, Celtic salt is a naturally harvested whole-crystal sea salt. It is produced today using the low-tech methods established in Brittany over two thousand years ago. This method allows Celtic salt to retain all of its minerals, electrolytes, and digestive enzymes that are beneficial to your health.
- Eat 100 percent whole-grain bread. This includes rye, spelt, wheat, barley, and oat. Some examples are Bread Alone Nine Mixed Grain bread and Ezekiel 4:9 Sprouted Whole Grain Bread. If you can't get 100 percent whole-grain bread, choose one that doesn't have preservatives or artificial flavors.
- In addition to the approved beverages in this book (see the Smoothies, Hot Drinks, and Juices section, page 32), the only other beverage you should consume during the Healing Phase is water. If you can't stand plain water, you can add cubes of watermelon to make the water slightly sweeter. Alternatively, you can add a few thin slices of cucumber to make the water more savory.
- When eating out, order chicken or seafood that is either steamed, roasted, baked, or grilled—never fried!

THE DOZEN FOOD *MYTHS* ABOUT THE ACID WATCHER DIET

Since the publication of The Acid Watcher Diet, *we are frequently faced with addressing some of the very confusing, often contradictory, information that is readily available online and in certain publications regarding the acidity or alkalinity of various foods. The purpose of this section is to highlight some of the more common myths that we encounter and to explain why these statements are not true.*

1

Start every day with lemon water.

WRONG!

Lemon is a very acidic substance and activates pepsin.

2

Apple cider vinegar (ACV) is a great natural treatment for acid reflux disease.

WRONG!

Vinegar, in any form, is very acidic and, like lemon water, will activate pepsin and cause body-wide inflammation. My patients generally report that their throat feels raw and very irritated when consuming ACV. While on rare occasions they have reported feeling some relief of heartburn with ACV, the price paid is a wave of swelling from stem to stern, or lips to chest.

3

Tomatoes are the best source of lycopenes, so I need to eat them for my health because I can't get lycopenes anywhere else.

NOT TRUE!

Lycopenes are among the most potent natural anti-inflammatory agents. However, there are better choices for lycopene that don't have the acidity of tomatoes. One of the best options is watermelon, which has a greater concentration of lycopenes per unit weight than tomatoes and is relatively alkaline.

4

You can never have raw tomatoes on the Acid Watcher Diet.

NO!

Most tomatoes have a pH ranging from 4.3 to 4.9, so raw tomatoes are okay to have in the Maintenance Phase of the Acid Watcher Diet. What one needs to be careful with is either tomato sauce or tomato paste, since invariably the sauces and pastes contain extremely acidic additives as well as carminatives such as onion and garlic.

5

You can change the pH of your blood by what you eat.

NO WAY!

Unless you have kidney failure, what you eat will never affect the pH of your blood. The body tightly regulates your acid base metabolism to keep the pH of your blood at 7.4.

6

Hard alcohol is worse than wine and beer for acid reflux sufferers.

NOT TRUE!

Wine, especially white and rosé, is very acidic (pH 3.3). Gin and vodkas that are potato based (Chopin, Spud, Long Island Vodka) and corn based (Tito's, Balls) are generally above pH 7, so they are much less acidic than wine and beer. As far as what mixers to use for these spirits, instead of acidic juices such as cranberry, grapefruit, or orange, liberally use ice with either cucumber slices or watermelon chunks.

7

Acid reflux sufferers can drink only plain water.

NO!

Watermelon and cucumber are excellent anti-inflammatory foods that can be added to water (see page 21).

8

Acid reflux sufferers should not consume berries.

NO!

"Naked" berries (blackberries, blueberries, strawberries, and raspberries) are indeed acidic. However, you can neutralize the acidity of berries in a smoothie with nondairy coconut, almond, rice, or non-GMO soy milk.

9

If you don't have heartburn, you don't have acid reflux.

NOT TRUE!

Acid reflux is not only about what comes up from the stomach but also what comes down from the mouth when one eats or drinks acidic substances. In fact, when one has a lot of acid reflux, the surrounding tissues of the stomach and esophagus become inflamed. And when these tissues are inflamed, they become numb, so you feel nothing. If you have had heartburn for a while and it suddenly "goes away," don't rejoice. Get yourself to a doctor to have your esophagus and stomach examined.

10

My doctor told me I need to have an "endoscopy" (a procedure that examines the esophagus, stomach, and small intestine), and that I would have to be sedated or knocked out for the procedure.

NOT TRUE!

There is a way to perform an endoscopy of the esophagus with the patient awake. It's called transnasal esophagoscopy, or TNE. In TNE, a thin camera (the size and softness of a piece of spaghetti) is placed via the nose to examine the throat and esophagus. By going through the nose—as opposed to going through the mouth, as is done during traditional exams of the esophagus—we can avoid the powerful gag reflex at the back of the throat.

11

Caffeine and chocolate are acidic.

NOT SO!

Caffeine and chocolate have a pH close to 6. Caffeine and chocolate have *physiological* effects that can cause inflammation, because they both loosen the lower esophageal sphincter and increase acid production by the stomach.

12

The Acid Watcher Diet is only useful if you have acid reflux disease.

NOT TRUE!

The Acid Watcher Diet helps relieve inflammation throughout the body, not just in the throat and esophagus.

THE pH VALUES of VARIOUS FOODS and BEVERAGES

RAW VEGETABLES and HERBS	
English cucumber	7.6
Cauliflower	7.2
Peas, sweet	6.8
Zucchini	6.8
Romaine lettuce	6.6
Spinach	6.5
Broccoli	6.28
Celery	6.24
Iceberg lettuce	6.23
Swiss chard	6.22
Asparagus	6.21
Cilantro	6.18
Kale	6.01
Cabbage	5.98
Arugula	5.92
Basil	5.92
Butternut squash	5.81
Parsley	5.65
Garden cucumber	5.44
Lemongrass	5.42
Bell pepper, orange	5.2
Bell pepper, green	4.8–5.89
Bell pepper, yellow	4.8–5.44
Bell pepper, red	4.8–5.24
Tomato, plum	4.51
Tomato, beefsteak	4.23
Tomato, grape or pearl	4.19

RAW and DRIED FRUITS	
Avocado	7.12
Watermelon	6.53
Cantaloupe	6.42
Persimmon, Fuyu	6.25
Lychee	5.91
Lemon zest	5.77
Banana	5.71
Pear, Asian	5.7
Papaya	5.66
Dates, Medjool or Deglet	5.49
Dragon fruit	5.45
Olives, green Cerignola (rinsed)	5.44
Olives, black Cerignola, in water	5.43
Honeydew	5.42
Olives, kalamata	5.4
Pumpkin	5.4
Orange zest	5.34
Lime zest	5.22
Pear, Bosc	5.15
Apricot, dried Turkish	5.1
Apple, Red Delicious	4.88
Kiwi	4.84
Mango	4.58
Fig	4.55
Apple, Golden Delicious	4.5
Cherries	4.43
Raisins (dark)	4.41
Apple, Gala	4.31
Prunes, dried	4.27
Peach, yellow	4.25
Pear, Forelle	4.2
Blueberries	4.19
Pear, Bartlett	4.15
Grapes, green seedless	4.12
Apple, dehydrated	4.05

ROOT VEGETABLES*

Mushroom, cremini	6.79
Potato, red skin (cooked)	6.4
Ginger	6.28
Leek	6.21
Beet	6.19
Garlic	6.17
Onion, sweet	6.15
Carrot	6.14
Potato, russet or Yukon Gold (cooked)	5.95
Sweet potato (cooked)	5.91
Carrot (cooked)	5.83
Beet (cooked)	5.79

*raw, unless otherwise specified

DAIRY PRODUCTS

Blue cheese	6.99
Butter (salted)	5.86
Cheese, hard (Dublin)	5.8
Cheese, hard (Parmesan)	5.4
Cheese, hard (Asiago)	5.2
Cheese, soft (mozzarella)	5.2
Cheese, hard (Cheddar)	5.16
Cottage cheese	4.64
Butter (unsalted)	4.63
Feta cheese	4.6
Cream cheese (Philadelphia)	4.59
Yogurt, plain (Stonyfield)	4.43
Yogurt, Greek, plain (Fage)	4.34
Goat cheese	4.32
Yogurt, Greek, plain (Chobani)	4.31
Kefir	4.17

EGGS

Egg white	8.84
Egg, hard-boiled	7.48
Egg yolk	6.32

DAIRY ALTERNATIVES

Almond milk, vanilla (Silk)	8.4
Almond milk, original flavor (Silk)	8.36
Almond milk (Califia Farms Organic Almond Homestyle Nutmilk, unsweetened)	7.9
Coconut milk (Califia Farms Go Coconuts Coconut milk)	7.6
Soy milk (Westsoy, unsweetened)	7.0
Tofu	6.9
Almond milk, homemade	6.62
Rice milk, plain	6.35
Almond yogurt, plain (Almond Dream)	4.67
Coconut milk yogurt, cultured, vanilla (So Delicious)	4.66
Soy yogurt, plain (WholeSoy & Co.)	4.64
Coconut milk yogurt, cultured, plain (So Delicious)	4.58
"Ricotta" cheese, dairy-free, (Kite Hill Almond Milk "Ricotta")	4.5
Soy yogurt, vanilla (WholeSoy & Co.)	4.44
Coconut milk yogurt, natural flavor (Coyo)	4.24
Coconut milk yogurt, plain (Anita's)	4.01

THE pH VALUES of VARIOUS FOODS and BEVERAGES

TREE NUTS

Almonds (raw)	6.08
Walnuts (raw)	5.96
Macadamia (raw)	5.48
Cashews (raw)	5.41
Hazelnuts (raw)	5.37
Pistachios (salted)	5.33

CONDIMENTS and SPREADS

Almond butter (natural)	6.32	Mayonnaise, egg-free (Primal Kitchen)	4.56
Peanut butter (freshly ground)	6.15	Soy sauce, less sodium (Kikkoman)	4.38
Maple syrup (Grade A, Amber Color and Rich Flavor)	6.06	Honey, manuka	4.31
Tahini, organic (Trader Joe's)	6.0	Capers (in salt)	4.27
Miso paste, organic (Ryotei No Aji by Marukome)	5.32	Agave nectar (light)	4.2
Sunflower seed butter, organic (Sunbutter)	5.3	Honey, raw	4.1
Vanilla extract, pure (Kirkland)	5.19	Coconut aminos seasoning sauce, organic (Trader Joe's)	3.82
Tamari	5.1	Mayonnaise (Hellman's)	3.8
Bragg's Liquid Aminos (soy sauce alternative)	5.0	Mustard (Gulden's spicy brown)	3.68
Vanilla extract, pure (Simply Organic Madagascar)	4.91	Vinegar, apple cider (Trader Joe's)	3.08
Soy sauce (Kikkoman)	4.82	Mustard, Dijon (Annie's)	3.1
Soy sauce, gluten- and preservative-free (Kikkoman)	4.69	Vinegar, white wine	2.96
		Vinegar, distilled white (Heinz)	2.52

WATER (UNFLAVORED, FLAT, and SPARKLING)

Essentia	9.53
Evamor	8.8
Aquadeco	7.78
Jana	7.78
Smart Water	7.7
Fiji	7.55
Evian	7.36
Arizona Vapor Water	7.3
NYC tap water (unfiltered)	7.23
NYC tap water (filtered)	6.81
Voss flat water	6.68
Perrier	5.64
Dasani	5.46
Distilled water	5.22
Pellegrino	5.03
LaCroix (plain, sparkling)	3.94

BEVERAGES (NONALCOHOLIC)

Pedialyte, unflavored (9 grams sugar)	5.52
Coconut water (Harmless Harvest)	5.4
Coconut water (Zico)	5.2
Pure Leaf unsweetened black tea	4.2
Monster energy drink	3.54
Red Bull	3.5
POM pomegranate juice	3.33
Gatorade glacier cherry (21 grams sugar)	3.32
Kombucha (GTS Enlightened Gingerade Raw, Organic)	3.12
Gatorade, lemon-lime (21 grams sugar)	3.06
Arizona Fruit Punch	2.98
Bai São Paolo strawberry lemonade	2.76
Nice! Tonic Water	2.71
Canada Dry Ginger Ale	2.7
Powerade Fruit Punch (21 grams sugar)	2.64

MEATS, POULTRY, FISH, and SHELLFISH

Lobster (boiled)	7.3
Shrimp (boiled)	6.92
Tilapia	6.8
Crabmeat	6.75
Monkfish	6.7
Halibut (poached)	6.62
Salmon (grilled)	6.32
Octopus (grilled)	6.3
Tuna (canned, in water)	6.18
Turkey (fresh, roasted)	6.17
Sardines (fresh)	6.15
Tuna (seared)	6.1
Cod (broiled)	6.05
Hamburger meat (cooked)	5.8
Chicken (grilled)	5.23
Beef (sirloin)	5.1

THE pH VALUES of VARIOUS FOODS and BEVERAGES

BREADS

Multigrain bread (Bread Alone Nine Mixed Grain bread)	5.53
Ezekiel 4:9 Flax Sprouted Grain Bread	5.48
100 percent whole-grain bread (Le Pain Quotidien)	5.35
Ezekiel 4:9 Sesame Sprouted Whole Grain Bread	5.27
Whole-wheat fiber bread (Mestemacher Natural Three Grain Bread)	5.07
Ezekiel 4:9 Cinnamon Raisin Sprouted Whole Grain Bread	4.64

LEGUMES

Peas, black-eyed	6.62
Edamame	6.57
Beans, cannellini, organic (canned, rinsed)	6.1
Chickpeas (Goya canned)	6.04
Beans, black (Goya canned)	5.93
Beans, red (Goya canned)	5.87

ALCOHOL

Note: Alcohol is not permitted during the Healing Phase, even if it is above pH 5.

BEER

Heineken	4.47
Bud Light	4.38
Stella Artois	4.26
Corona Extra	4.21
Coors Light	4.1

BITTERS

Breckinridge	5.16

BRANDY

Germain-Robin	3.87
Rodin Napoleon	3.57

CACHAÇA

Pitu	4.4
51	4.34

CHAMPAGNE

Nicolas Feuillatte	3.26

GIN

Cold River (Maine)	7.73
Greenhook Ginsmiths	7.3

LIQUEUR

Grand Marnier	4.06

PROSECCO

Mionetto Brut	3.28

ROCK & RYE

Mister Katz	4.59

RUM

Lost Spirits (Monterey, California)	5.03
Old New Orleans	4.48
Gosling's Black Seal Black	4.06
Bacardi Reserva Limitada Puerto Rican	3.8

SAKE

Gekkeikan	4.38

SAMBUCA

Romana	4.27

SCOTCH

Johnnie Walker Black	4.25
Oban	4.09
Balvenie	3.98
Glenrothes	3.88

TEQUILA

Corzo Silver	6.15
Don Julio Reposado	4.78
Don Julio Real Añejo	4.6
Partida Reposado	4.38
Patrón Silver	4.21
Partida Añejo	4.2
Chinaco Blanco	4.19
Jose Cuervo Reserva de la Familia	4.05

VERMOUTH

Atsby	3.69

VODKA
(grain-based unless otherwise stated)

Chopin (potato)	8.69
Industry Standard	8.1
Tito (corn)	7.8
Pinnacle	7.78
Beluga	7.44
Absolut	7.26
Grey Goose Orange	6.03

WHISKEY

Breckinridge	4.4
Zeppelin Bend	4.13

WINE

Red

Pinot Noir	
Leese-Fitch, California 2016	3.68
Merlot	
Jacob's Creek, Australia 2016	3.53
Cabernet Sauvignon	
Excelsior, South Africa 2016	3.48

Rosé

Maison Marcel, France 2017	3.24

White

Chardonnay	
Sanford, Santa Barbara 2007	3.49
Sauvignon Blanc	
Indaba, South Africa 2016	3.38
Pinot Grigio	
Danzante, Italy 2016	3.36

THE RECIPES

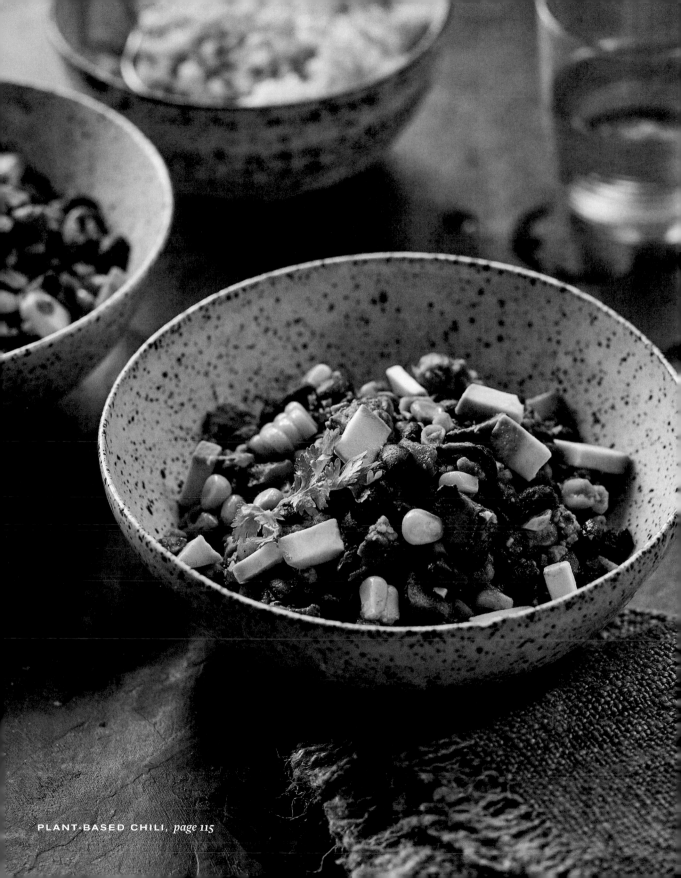

PLANT-BASED CHILI, *page 115*

SMOOTHIES, HOT DRINKS, and JUICES

H   HEALING PHASE   M   MAINTENANCE PHASE

"PB&J" Basic
BERRY SMOOTHIE

SERVES 2
Prep Time: 5 minutes

---

1 medium ripe banana
2 cups fresh or frozen mixed berries
2 tablespoons organic peanut butter
   or almond butter
1 cup soy milk or almond milk

The simple, satisfying, and not-so-healthy peanut butter and jelly (PB&J) sandwich is updated and made healthier in this nut butter and mixed-berry smoothie.

Combine all the ingredients in a blender and blend until smooth. Pour into glasses and enjoy.

KITCHEN NOTE 1   We want to share an important preparation tip for those using a Vitamix blender. With recipes using small volumes of ingredients (less than 2 cups), use one with a 3-inch base. If you use a Vitamix with a 4-inch base, the ingredients will not mix properly, but will instead collect, unmixed, under the cutting blades of the blender.

KITCHEN NOTE 2   In the ingredient lists where fruits and vegetables are listed, unless stated otherwise, they are unpeeled—except, of course, for the banana.

BEET BERRY SMOOTHIE

SERVES 2
Prep Time: 10 minutes

---

1 cup peeled and chopped raw beets
½ cup fresh or frozen blackberries
½ cup fresh or frozen raspberries
1 cup soy milk

We were initially concerned that a beet-based smoothie might sound like an awful-tasting concoction. It is actually a delicious Healing Phase recipe.

Combine all the ingredients in a blender and blend until smooth. Pour into glasses and enjoy.

DOCTOR'S NOTE The concept of neutralizing acidic foods with alkaline foods is embodied in smoothies, where very acidic fruits, such as berries and even citrus, are neutralized with certain concentrated alkaline liquids (*not* water). I like to use the acronym CARS as a reminder that nondairy "milks" such as coconut, almond, rice, and soy milks are ideal neutralizers. So you can preserve the antioxidant effect of various acidic fruits while taking away the inflammatory effects of their acidity. Additionally, you can use alkaline fruits and vegetables, such as several types of melon and zucchini, which will also raise the pH. The CARS "milks" used in the recipes are all unflavored and unsweetened.

GOLDEN DELISH SMOOTHIE

SERVES 2

Prep Time: 5 minutes

2 Gala or Golden Delicious apples, cored
1 (½-inch) piece fresh ginger, peeled, single piece
¼ cup old-fashioned rolled oats
1 tablespoon flaxseeds
¼ teaspoon ground cinnamon
1 cup nondairy milk

While the banana is a staple of many a smoothie, we sought to create a fruit-based smoothie without a banana, using rolled oats to thicken the beverage. This is a Maintenance Phase (i.e., above pH 4) smoothie because it uses raw cinnamon, which loosens the lower esophageal muscle.

Combine all the ingredients in a blender and blend until smooth. Pour into glasses and enjoy.

Honeydew Pear
GINGER SMOOTHIE

SERVES 2
Prep Time: 5 minutes

---

1 medium ripe banana
2 cups 1-inch cubed honeydew melon
1 Bosc pear, cored
1 (½- to 1-inch) piece fresh ginger, peeled, single piece
2 cups almond milk
Handful of ice (optional)

The combined alkalinity of melon, banana, and almond milk essentially allows the addition of almost any fruit to this smoothie to keep it above pH 5, therefore making it Healing Phase–friendly. Adding a Bosc pear and some fresh ginger spices things up.

Combine all the ingredients in a blender and blend until smooth. Pour into glasses and enjoy.

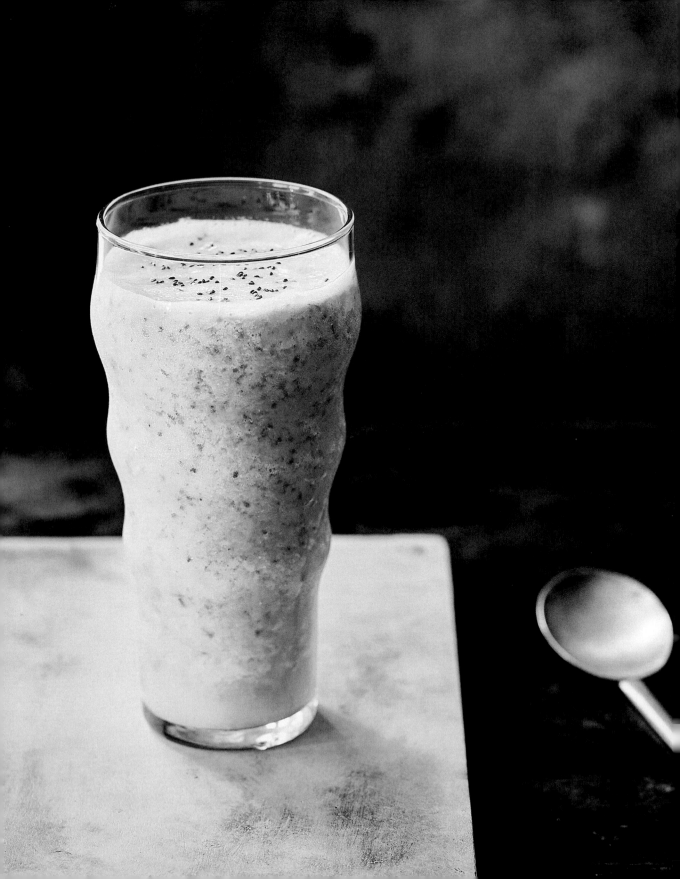

ORANGE CREAM SMOOTHIE

SERVES 2
Prep Time: 5 minutes

1 medium ripe banana
1 navel orange, peeled and halved
1 tablespoon flax- or chia seeds
1 cup soy milk or almond milk
1 cup ice

Missing your morning citrus? We have neutralized the highly acidic orange with relatively alkaline "milk" to create a tangy and refreshing smoothie for those on the Maintenance Phase. This is an Acid Watcher–safe way of using citrus to start your day.

Combine all the ingredients in a blender and blend until smooth. Pour into glasses and enjoy.

PIÑA KALEADA SMOOTHIE

SERVES 2
Prep Time: 5 minutes

---

2 medium ripe bananas
1 cup frozen pineapple chunks
2 cups chopped curly kale
2 tablespoons unsweetened
 shredded coconut
2 cups soy milk

Dreaming of a tropical getaway? Then this smoothie is for you. Don't have coconut milk around? No worries—be happy—we've made it easy for you by subbing shredded coconut for the coconut milk. Shredded coconut gives this smoothie the texture of a fresh coconut-based mocktail, without the unwanted fat, calories, and preservatives found in traditional beach beverages. The strong, fruity flavor of pineapple overpowers the kale, leaving you with a healthy, refreshing, *and* nutritious treat. This is surely a summer (or winter!) morning, noon, or nighttime fave.

Note that the pineapple acidity is neutralized by the alkalinity of nut milk, kale, and coconut.

Combine all the ingredients in a blender and blend until smooth. Pour into glasses and enjoy.

CHAWCOLATE HAZELNUT SHAKE

SERVES 2
Prep Time: 5 minutes

2 medium ripe bananas
⅓ cup old-fashioned rolled oats
2 tablespoons carob powder
⅔ cup raw shelled hazelnuts
2 cups almond milk

We capture the delicious but inflammatory combination of hazelnut, chocolate, milk, and processed sugar typically found in chocolate hazelnut sweets with this dairy-free and processed sugar–free treat. Carob powder and almond milk substitute for chocolate and cow's milk, respectively.

Combine all the ingredients in a blender and blend until smooth. Pour into glasses and enjoy.

KEY LIME PIE SMOOTHIE

SERVES 2
Prep time: 5 minutes

---

2 frozen medium ripe bananas
 (peel before freezing)
2 cups packed fresh baby spinach
Zest of 2 limes
2 tablespoons fresh lime juice
2 Deglet dates, pitted
2 cups soy milk

This refreshing, oh-so-citrusy lime-based smoothie is Healing Phase–friendly.

Combine all the ingredients in a blender and blend until smooth. Pour into glasses and enjoy.

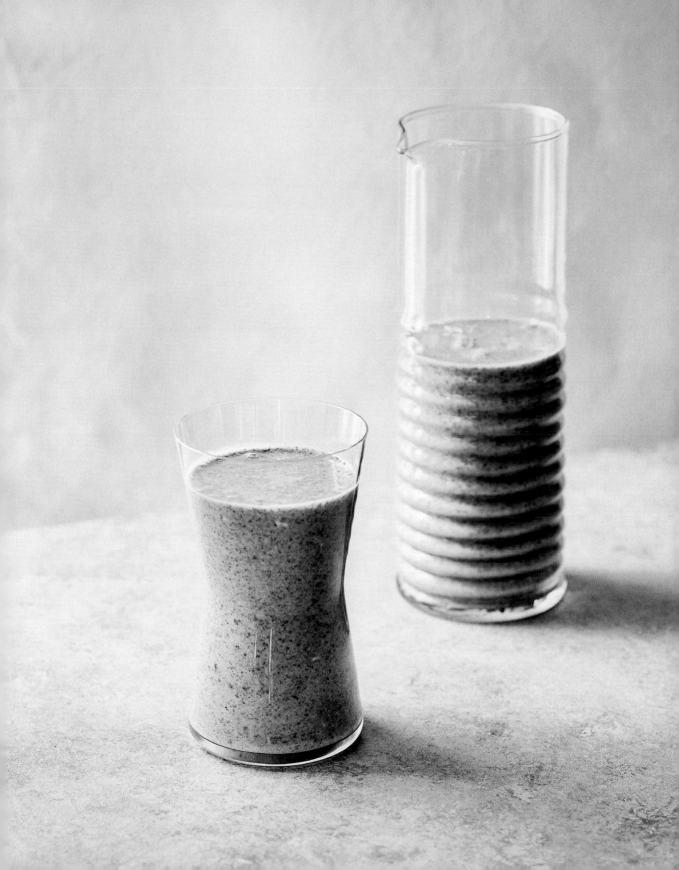

PUMPKIN PIE SMOOTHIE

SERVES 2

Prep Time: 5 minutes

2 frozen medium ripe bananas (peel before freezing)

1 cup organic pumpkin puree

2 tablespoons dark raisins

2 cups almond milk

Dash of ground cinnamon

As soon as there's a nip in the air, people start developing a craving for everything pumpkin. This smoothie is the perfect pumpkin-craving killer. The minute amount of raw cinnamon makes it safe for those on the Maintenance Phase of the diet. Since you're already in the Maintenance Phase, dare to be wild and add an extra dash of cinnamon.

Combine all the ingredients in a blender and blend until smooth. Pour into glasses and enjoy.

TURMERIC LATTE

SERVES 2
Prep and Cook Time: 10 minutes

2 cups soy milk
1 (1-inch) piece fresh ginger, peeled, single piece
½ teaspoon ground cinnamon
¼ teaspoon ground turmeric
1 tablespoon raw honey

Heating spices such as cinnamon and turmeric effectively dampens their carminative effect. Turmeric has antioxidant and therefore anti-inflammatory properties, primarily as a result of its active ingredient, curcumin.

1   In a small saucepan set over medium heat, combine the soy milk and ginger and bring to a simmer. Do not boil!

2   Add the spices and honey, and whisk continuously for 2 to 3 minutes. Turn off the heat, remove the ginger, pour into mugs, and enjoy.

DOCTOR'S NOTE   When you're missing that morning cup of joe in the Healing Phase, this recipe and those on pages 46 and 47 are a few alternatives. Remember that while coffee is not acidic, it has the "double whammy" physiologic effect of loosening the lower esophageal muscle and increasing acid production by the stomach, but it is not going to activate tissue-bound pepsin in the mouth and throat.

Chicory and Vanilla
CAFFEINE-FREE LATTE

SERVES 2

Prep and Cook Time: 10 minutes, plus an overnight soak for the cashews

---

½ cup raw unsalted cashews, soaked in water overnight

2¾ cups filtered water

1 tablespoon ground chicory

2 tablespoons manuka honey

½ teaspoon pure vanilla extract

If you're sensitive to the effects of caffeine—be it heartburn, heart racing, sweating, irritable bowel, or a combination thereof (how's that for a stressful morning?)—you can use chicory as an alternative to capture some of the flavor of coffee without its physiological consequences.

Chicory is a plant, but it is the *root* of the plant that is used in food. Because of its woody, nutty taste once it is roasted and ground, it can be used as either a coffee extender or a coffee substitute. Numerous retailers carry ground chicory.

1   In a blender, combine the cashews, after they are rinsed and drained, and ¾ cup of the water and puree until completely smooth, about 1 minute. Set the cashew "milk" aside.

2   In a 1½-quart saucepan over high heat, bring the remaining 2 cups water to a boil. Stir in the chicory and remove from the heat.

3   Divide the hot chicory "coffee" between two mugs. To each, add ¼ cup cashew milk, 1 tablespoon manuka honey, and ¼ teaspoon vanilla, and stir. Serve.

Ginger, Pear, and Manuka HONEY "CIDER"

SERVES 2
Prep and Cook Time: 25 minutes

1 (2-inch) piece fresh ginger, peeled and sliced
1 Bosc pear, cored and sliced into sixths
1 tablespoon manuka honey (optional)
2 cups water

The cider house rules! This Acid Watcher Healing Phase cider uses fresh ginger to tang up the Bosc pear while keeping the pH above 5.

In a small saucepan over high heat, combine the sliced ginger, pear, and honey (if using) with the water, and boil for at least 20 minutes, reducing the heat as necessary to prevent the liquid from spilling over the pot. Stir until the honey is fully dissolved. Remove the ginger and pear slices, pour into mugs, and serve.

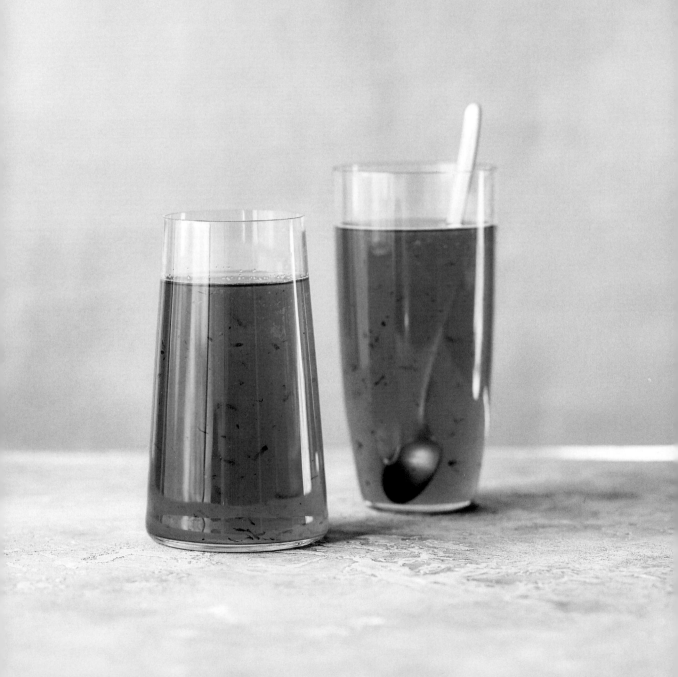

Watermelon Cucumber JUICE

SERVES 2
Prep Time: 5 minutes

1½ cups 1-inch cubed seedless watermelon
1 cup sliced English cucumber
Handful of ice
1 tablespoon flaxseeds (optional; see Note)

Many people believe that tomatoes have the highest concentration of lycopene, which is a powerful natural anti-inflammatory agent. This is why men often hear from their doctors that tomatoes are good for prostate health. However, pound for pound or milligram for milligram, watermelon has the greatest concentration of lycopenes, and it is not acidic. Joining the anti-inflammatory brigade is cucumber, which has a high concentration of lignan, also a powerful anti-inflammatory agent. The two in combination not only taste delicious but also pack a powerful anti-inflammatory wallop, something we call "food steroids."

Combine all the ingredients in a blender (see Doctor's Note) and blend until smooth. Pour into glasses and enjoy.

DOCTOR'S NOTE The juices in the Acid Watcher Diet are *blended* in a blender, not juiced in a juicer. Juicing often eliminates fiber, which can help reduce inflammation. It's important to retain as much fiber as possible.

NOTE To provide even more anti-inflammatory agents to this beverage, add 1 tablespoon flaxseeds, which contain a large amount of lignans.

Beet Apple Ginger
JUICE

SERVES 2
Prep Time: 5 minutes

1 (¼-inch) piece fresh ginger, peeled, single piece
1 cup peeled and chopped raw beets
1 Fuji apple, cored and sliced
2 cups ice cubes

Fun with raw beets continues, as the ginger gives a spicy kick to this juice. The beet and ginger combine to neutralize the acidity of the Fuji apple.

Combine all the ingredients in a blender and blend until smooth. Pour into glasses and enjoy.

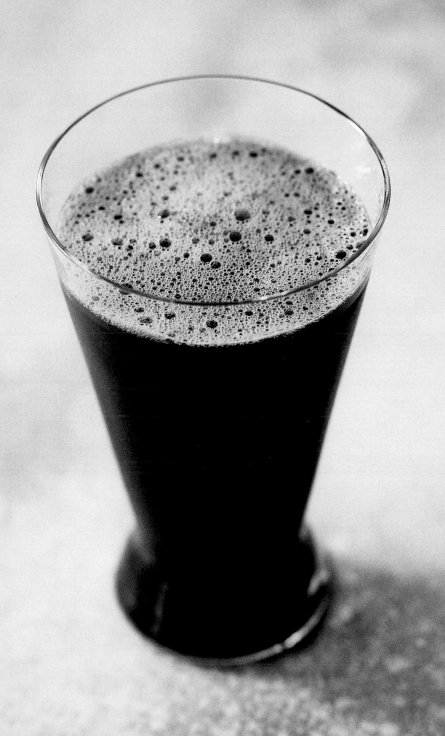

RISE AND SHINE BREAKFASTS

H HEALING PHASE   M MAINTENANCE PHASE

Creamy Herb-Infused FRITTATA

SERVES 4
Prep and Cook Time: 35 minutes

---

2 tablespoons olive oil, plus more if needed

3 cups chopped kale leaves

4 ounces firm tofu, cut into small pieces, about 2 inches or so

8 large eggs

½ teaspoon coarsely ground Celtic salt

⅓ cup soy milk

¼ cup finely chopped fresh herb leaves, preferably parsley or cilantro

2 scallions, white and green parts, chopped, or 1 tablespoon chopped chives (optional for Maintenance Phase)

A frittata is an open omelet cooked on the stovetop and finished in the oven. The most obvious difference between these dishes is that the omelet is served folded whereas the frittata is sliced and served. The texture and taste of the frittata can be enhanced by additional favorites—such as kale and tofu—and enjoyed any time of day. Any variety of kale will do for this recipe, but if you are not using the bagged, prechopped, and prewashed variety, make sure you remove and discard the stem and chop the leaves coarsely. Serve this with a side of lignan-laden, alkaline cucumbers and Real Hummus (page 87). For a more aromatic frittata, whisk your favorite finely chopped fresh herbs, such as parsley or cilantro, into the egg mixture. In the Maintenance Phase you can also add chives or scallions.

1   Preheat the oven to 350°F. Position one rack slightly above the center.

2   Heat the oil in a nonstick, ovenproof skillet over medium-low heat. Add the kale and sauté for 5 to 7 minutes, until it wilts, adding up to 2 tablespoons water, if needed, to prevent sticking. Once the kale has wilted, add the tofu and sauté for another 2 minutes. Spread the kale and tofu evenly in a single layer.

3   While the kale and tofu sauté, in a separate bowl whisk the eggs, salt, and soy milk. Stir in the herbs and, if using, the scallions or chives. Pour the egg mixture over the kale and tofu. Reduce the heat to low and cover the pan. Cook for about 5 minutes, or until the edge of the frittata begins to crisp.

4   Remove the cover and place the skillet into the oven. Bake for 3 minutes.

5   Turn on the broiler for about another 2 minutes, or until the top of the frittata begins to char. Remove the frittata from the oven and cool for at least 5 to 10 minutes before serving. Serve warm.

TOFU SCRAMBLE

SERVES 2

Prep and Cook Time: 20 minutes

---

2 teaspoons olive oil
6 button mushrooms, sliced
1 teaspoon finely ground Celtic salt
1 (14-ounce) block firm tofu, rinsed
¼ teaspoon ground turmeric
¼ teaspoon sweet paprika
3 tablespoons almond milk or other
    nondairy milk
1 cup baby spinach

For those desiring a savory plant-based start to your day, this Healing Phase–friendly tofu scramble hits the spot.

1 In a medium pan over medium-high heat, warm 1 teaspoon of the olive oil and add the sliced mushrooms in an even layer. Sprinkle with ¼ teaspoon of the salt and sauté for 5 minutes, stirring occasionally. Transfer to a plate and set aside.

2 Pat the tofu with a paper towel to remove excess moisture.

3 In the same pan that you cooked the mushrooms, warm the remaining 1 teaspoon olive oil over medium-high heat. Crumble in the tofu by hand and season with the remaining ¾ teaspoon salt. Cook for 4 minutes, stirring occasionally. Stir in the turmeric and paprika and let cook for another minute until fragrant. Pour in the almond milk and cook for another minute, then remove from the heat.

4 Stir in the cooked mushrooms and the baby spinach. Plate and serve.

HUEVOS RANCHEROS

SERVES 2
Prep and Cook Time: 20 minutes

2 corn tortillas, preferably Trader Joe's Corn Tortillas or Ezekiel 4:9 Sprouted Corn Tortillas
1 (15-ounce) can black beans
¼ teaspoon ground cumin
¾ teaspoon finely ground Celtic salt
1 teaspoon lime zest
½ teaspoon olive oil
2 large eggs
1 ripe avocado, peeled, pitted, and cubed
Pico de Gallo (page 83)

The trace of lime in the corn tortilla unlocks essential amino acids in the corn that would otherwise remain unavailable to us.

1   Preheat the oven to 350°F. Place the corn tortillas on a baking sheet and bake until crispy and fragrant, about 10 minutes, flipping once halfway through.

2   In the meantime, add the whole can of black beans and the liquid into a small saucepan set over medium heat. Stir in the cumin and ¼ teaspoon of the salt. Bring to a simmer and cook for 5 minutes. Add the lime zest, stir, and set aside.

3   Heat the olive oil over medium heat in a separate skillet. Crack 2 eggs in and sprinkle each egg with ¼ teaspoon of salt. Let cook for about 3 minutes, until the whites set and the bottoms turn slightly golden brown. Gently flip the eggs and cook for an additional 2 minutes.

4   Place one crispy corn tortilla on each plate and top it with half the warm, saucy black beans, an egg, avocado, and some pico de gallo. Serve.

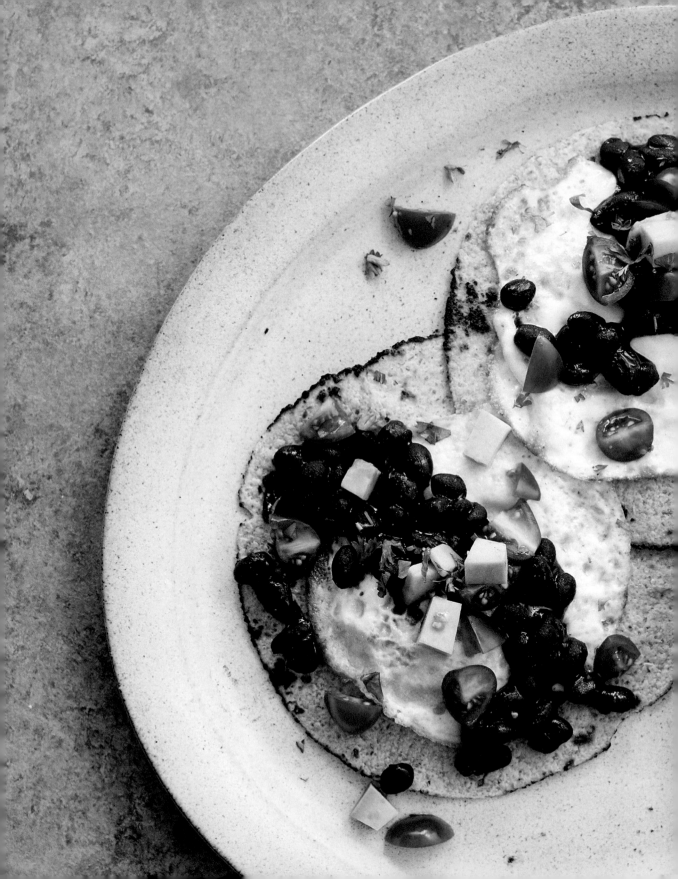

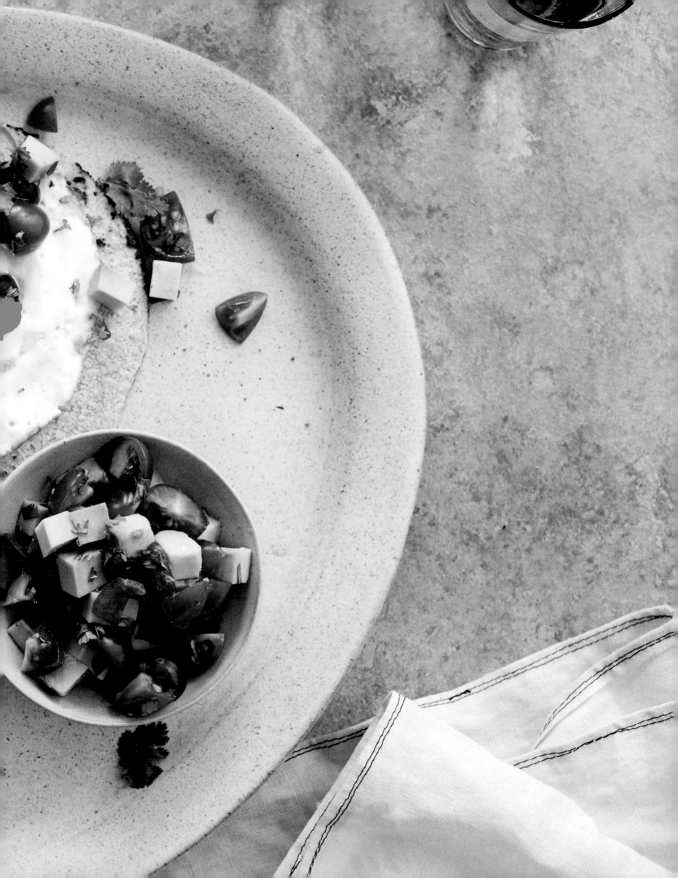

Cauliflower
TOSTADAS

MAKES TWELVE 5-INCH TOSTADAS
Prep and Cook Time: 50 minutes,
plus cooling time
(30 minutes in the freezer
or 1 to 2 hours in the refrigerator)

Cauliflower florets, 1 to 1½ pounds
1⅔ cups masa harina
1 teaspoon coarsely ground Celtic salt
½ teaspoon Mexican oregano
½ teaspoon ground coriander
1 large egg
1 to 2 tablespoons olive oil

This gluten-free version of tostadas is packed with fiber and nutrients, thanks to the cauliflower. You can use it as a base for more classic taco ingredients such as shredded chicken, beans, cabbage, or guacamole, or as a simple egg breakfast, as in Acid Watcher Eggs Benedict (aka Green Eggs Without Ham) (page 62). You can enjoy the tostada as a snack with just about any Acid Watcher–approved condiment. Make it casual (with hummus and sprouts) or super fancy (with hard-boiled eggs and caviar). Just remember that without gluten, the tostadas are fragile, so handle with care.

1   Fill a 2-quart saucepan halfway with water and bring to a boil over high heat.

2   In the meantime, wash the cauliflower florets and, using your fingers, break them into small pieces, 1 to 2 inches in size. Pulse in a large food processor— in two batches if necessary—5 to 7 seconds at a time until the florets are reduced to a pebble-like consistency. Stop occasionally to scrape the cauliflower from the sides of the processor and reintegrate it into the mixture. Don't overprocess the mixture or the cauliflower will become soupy.

3   Transfer the pulsed cauliflower florets to the pot of boiling water, reduce the heat to medium-low, and simmer, stirring occasionally, for 5 to 7 minutes, until the florets soften. Using a fine-mesh sieve, drain the cauliflower and immediately rinse it with cold water (let it run for 60 to 90 seconds) until the cauliflower fully cools. Drain again, squeezing out any excess water. (Give it 15 to 20 squeezes by hand; it should look like mashed potatoes after you are done.) Set aside.

4　In a large bowl, whisk the masa harina, salt, oregano, and coriander. Add the cooked cauliflower and 1 cup water to the masa and spice mix. Blend thoroughly using a wooden or a silicone spoon.

5　Whisk in the egg and 1 tablespoon of oil and stir to thoroughly combine. If the dough seems to be too dry, add another tablespoon of oil. The dough should be thick and pull away from the sides of the bowl.

6　Line a cutting board with plastic wrap. Transfer the dough and form it into a log about 4 inches in diameter and 6 inches long. Wrap in plastic wrap and refrigerate for 1 to 2 hours, or 30 minutes in the freezer.

7　To bake the tostadas, preheat the oven to 425°F. Line a large baking sheet with parchment paper.

8　Unwrap the log and place it on a cutting board. Cut the log evenly into 12 disks and flatten each slightly with your hands to 5 inches or so in diameter. Carefully transfer the disks to the lined baking sheet. Make sure you leave enough space, at least ½ inch, between each disk to allow you to flip them.

9　Bake for 20 minutes, carefully flipping the tostadas halfway through the baking process. Remove from the oven when the outer edges of the tostadas are crispy and lightly browned. Serve immediately.

ACID WATCHER EGGS BENEDICT
(*aka Green Eggs Without Ham*)

SERVES 6

Prep and Cook Time: 10 to 15 minutes

You'll never miss the acid trigger bomb of English muffin, Canadian bacon, and Hollandaise sauce in this inventive take on the classic eggs Benedict.

2 tablespoons olive oil
12 large eggs
12 Cauliflower Tostadas (page 60)
Electric Green Goddess Dressing (page 169)
12 (1-ounce) slices smoked salmon, one for each tostada
Celtic salt (optional)

1   Preheat the oil in a large nonstick pan over high heat. Crack the eggs, one at a time, and place them into the pan. (If you are using a small pan, we recommend frying two eggs at a time, using ½ teaspoon of oil per egg.) Lower the heat and cook for 2 minutes. If you prefer your yolks to be fully cooked, cover the pan for another minute. Remove from the heat.

2   Place 2 tostadas on each serving plate. Dollop approximately 2 tablespoons of the Electric Green Goddess Dressing in the center of each tostada, and spread it around with the back of a spoon. Layer with the salmon and egg on top. Sprinkle with salt, if desired, and serve immediately.

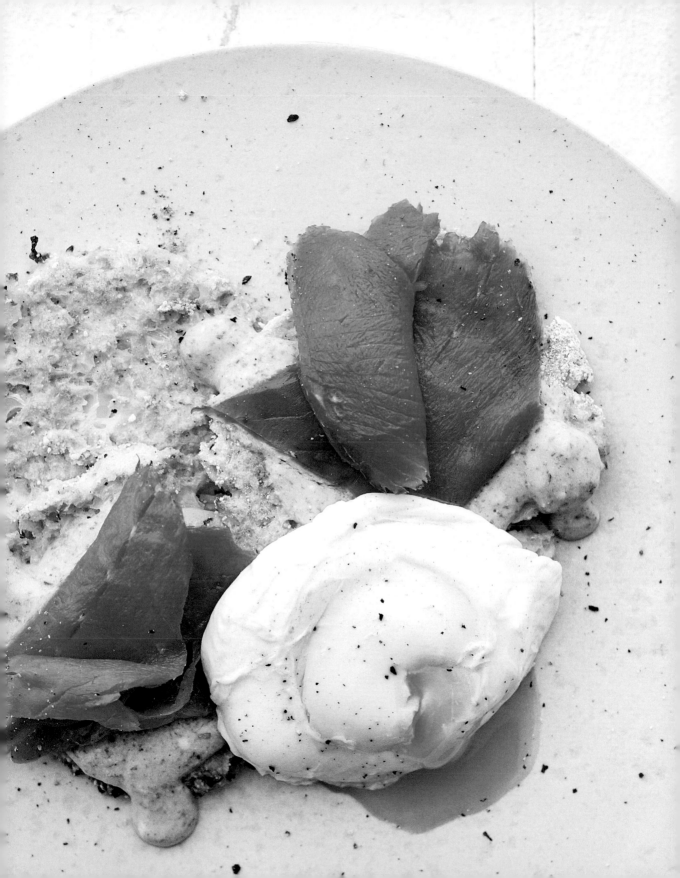

Banana Blender PANCAKES

SERVES 2;
MAKES FOUR 3- TO 4-INCH
PANCAKES
Prep and Cook Time: 10 minutes

1 cup old-fashioned rolled oats
2 large eggs
4 large egg whites
2 medium ripe bananas
1 teaspoon baking powder
Pinch of coarsely ground Celtic salt
1 teaspoon olive oil or organic butter
   (unsalted)
Raw Date Syrup (page 177),
   Berry Jam (page 179), or Apple
   and Pear Sauce (page 82), for
   serving (optional; see Note)

Even "healthy" prepackaged pancake mixes are processed and not a healthy option when the craving strikes for fluffy pancakes morning, noon, or night. Furthermore, to make them palatable, you have to douse them in syrup, which adds a copious amount of calories and sugar. These Acid Watcher–friendly pancakes are as easy to make as the prepackaged mixes and are naturally sweetened with banana to cut back on the need for extra sweeteners. To add a bit more sweetness and festiveness, pair these with our Raw Date Syrup, Berry Jam, or Apple and Pear Sauce.

1   Combine the oats, eggs, egg whites, bananas, baking powder, and salt in a blender and blend on high until the mixture is smooth and resembles a traditional pancake batter (approximately 1 minute).

2   Heat a large nonstick pan over medium-high heat. Using a pastry brush, grease the pan with the oil.

3   Pour approximately one-quarter of the batter directly into the pan to form each pancake, 3 to 4 inches in diameter, and reduce the heat to medium. Once bubbles form, carefully flip the pancakes and cook for another 60 to 90 seconds until the underside is golden brown.

4   Transfer to plates and, if desired, top with raw date syrup, berry jam, or apple and pear sauce. Serve.

NOTE   Using Berry Jam and/or Apple and Pear Sauce will make this a Maintenance Phase dish.

Gluten-Free
OAT WAFFLES

**MAKES TWO OR THREE 8-INCH
WAFFLES**
Prep and Cook Time: 30 minutes

2 cups oat flour
2 teaspoons baking powder
2 teaspoons raw honey
1 teaspoon pure vanilla extract
1 cup soy milk
1 large egg
2 large egg whites
1½ teaspoons coconut oil, melted

Traditional Belgian waffles are devoid of any nutritional value and filled with refined carbohydrates and processed sugar. Meet the Acid Watcher waffle, whose ingredients are almost identical to those in a bowl of oatmeal, but that tastes just like a traditional fluffy diner, drive-in, and dive waffle. We prefer the stainless steel Black + Decker Belgian Waffle Maker; your cooking time may be different if you have a different brand.

1   In a blender, combine the oat flour, baking powder, honey, vanilla, soy milk, egg, and egg whites, and blend until smooth, approximately 2 minutes. Let the batter rest and thicken for 10 minutes.

2   Preheat the waffle iron and brush each side with ½ teaspoon of the coconut oil.

3   When the waffle iron is ready, add approximately 1 cup of the batter, close, and cook for 8 to 10 minutes, or until the waffle is golden brown. Remove from the waffle iron and keep warm. Repeat with the remaining batter, brushing both sides of the waffle iron each time with the coconut oil.

4   Serve immediately or store the waffles between parchment paper in the freezer for up to 2 weeks. Reheat them as needed in the toaster.

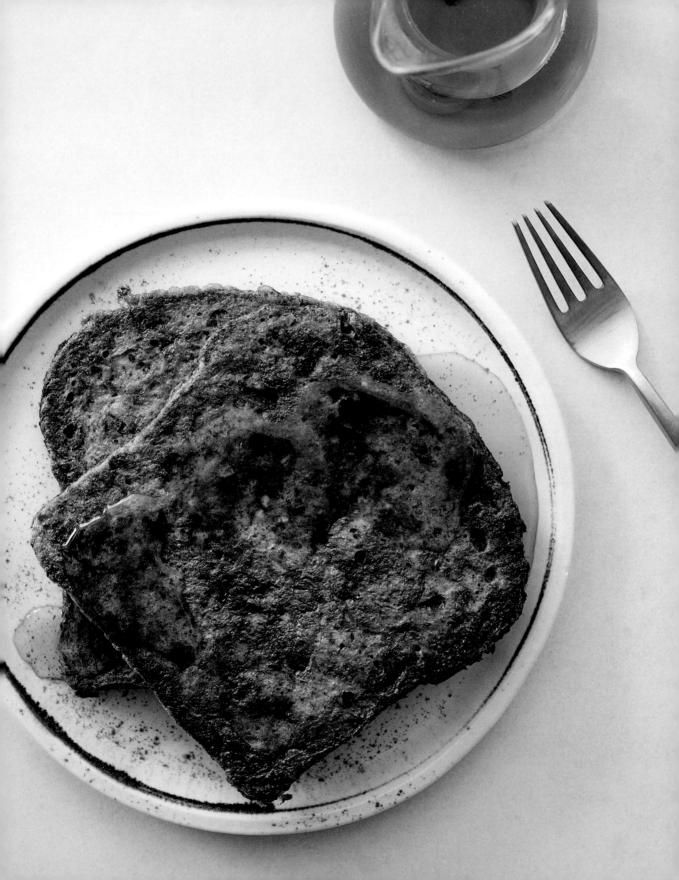

Cinnamon Raisin
FRENCH TOAST

SERVES 2; MAKES 4 SLICES

Prep and Cook Time: 15 minutes

---

4 large eggs

2 teaspoons pure vanilla extract

¼ cup almond milk

4 teaspoons ground cinnamon

4 slices Ezekiel 4:9 Cinnamon Raisin
Sprouted Whole Grain Bread,
thawed

1 to 2 teaspoons coconut oil, melted

4 teaspoons pure maple syrup
or Raw Date Syrup (page 177),
for serving (optional)

Had enough waffles? This version of French toast features cinnamon-raisin Ezekiel bread and uses almond milk to neutralize the vestiges of acidity brought in by the raisins. The cooking process dampens the carminative effect of the cinnamon while maintaining its distinctive flavor.

1   Combine the eggs, vanilla, almond milk, and cinnamon in a large, shallow baking dish and whisk to combine thoroughly.

2   Soak the bread, 2 slices at a time, in the egg mixture for 45 seconds on each side.

3   Heat 1 teaspoon of the oil in a large nonstick pan over medium-high heat. Transfer the soaked bread to the pan, reduce the heat to medium, and cook for 3 to 4 minutes on the first side until golden brown. Flip and cook for another 1 to 2 minutes, or until golden brown on both sides.

4   Serve immediately, with syrup, if desired.

Mediterranean
BANANA
BREAD

SERVES 10 TO 12

Prep and Cook Time: 1 hour 5 minutes

⅓ cup olive oil, plus more for the pan

⅓ cup raw honey

2 large eggs

3 medium overripe bananas, peeled and mashed

2 tablespoons unsweetened applesauce

¼ cup almond milk, preferably homemade (page 190)

1 teaspoon baking soda

½ teaspoon coarsely ground Celtic salt

½ teaspoon ground cinnamon

1 teaspoon pure vanilla extract

1¾ cups whole-wheat flour

½ cup chopped walnuts

This bread is such a treat that you will likely find yourself eating it throughout the day, both as a snack and as a dessert! We've swapped the butter for olive oil, drastically cutting the saturated fat found in traditional banana bread without detracting from the taste. Plus, it's 100 percent whole wheat, filling and satisfying, and not bitter or grainy. We recommend using the Copper Chef Loaf Pan that has a "lift and serve" insert for ease and convenience. It allows quick and simple removal of the bread without having to line a loaf pan.

1   Preheat the oven to 350°F. Brush a 9 × 5 × 3-inch loaf pan with a small amount of olive oil and set it aside.

2   In a large bowl, beat the ⅓ cup oil and honey together with a whisk. Add the eggs and whisk. Add the mashed bananas, applesauce, and almond milk, and mix together. Add the baking soda, salt, cinnamon, and vanilla, and continue whisking. With a large spoon, stir in the flour to incorporate. Gently fold in the walnuts, and pour the batter into the prepared loaf pan.

3   Bake for about 55 minutes, or until a toothpick inserted into the middle of the loaf comes out clean. Let cool, remove the bread, slice, and serve. Store leftovers, covered, in the fridge for up to 2 days.

BLACK CHERRY YOGURT

SERVES 2

Prep Time: 5 minutes,
plus 20 to 30 minutes for thawing

⅔ cup frozen dark sweet cherries
1 (5.3-ounce) container unsweetened
   nondairy coconut "milk" yogurt
   (about ½ cup)
1 teaspoon raw honey (optional)

Yogurt, plain or fruit flavored, is often a go-to "healthy snack." However, dairy yogurt can be inflammatory due to the casein found in cow's milk–based foods, and the relatively acidic pH of unflavored yogurt is typically around 4.1. Once any type of flavoring is added to the yogurt, the amount of sugar soars, and the entire mixture typically drops below 4.0, so it is quite acidic in addition to its sugar load. The Acid Watcher version of fruit-flavored yogurt uses nondairy, unsweetened coconut yogurt.

1   Thaw the cherries by letting them sit at room temperature for 20 to 30 minutes; they should still be very cold but not frozen solid.

2   Place the cherries in the bowl of a food processor and puree until smooth.

3   Divide the yogurt and the cherry puree between two small bowls. You can enjoy the puree on the bottom, side, or top of your yogurt, or mix it in fully. If you enjoy a sweeter treat, stir the honey into the mixture.

Lemon Blueberry
CHIA PUDDING

SERVES 2

Prep Time: 10 minutes,
plus 6 to 12 hours for chilling

1 cup soy milk
Zest of 1 lemon
1 tablespoon fresh lemon juice
1 teaspoon pure vanilla extract
1 tablespoon manuka honey
2 tablespoons chia seeds
½ cup fresh blueberries

Thanks to the acidity-neutralizing food science of the Acid Watcher concepts, we are able to use traditionally very acidic fresh citrus fruit in preparing this dairy-free morning chia pudding. Even the acidic dash of lemon juice is neutralized by the precise combination of non-GMO soy milk and chia seeds.

1   In a medium bowl, preferably one with a pour spout, whisk together the soy milk, lemon zest and juice, vanilla, and honey until well combined.

2   Add the chia seeds and whisk to combine thoroughly. Pour the mixture into two airtight 6-ounce jars, cover, and refrigerate for at least 6 hours or up to overnight.

3   Once the pudding is done chilling, top each jar with half the blueberries and enjoy.

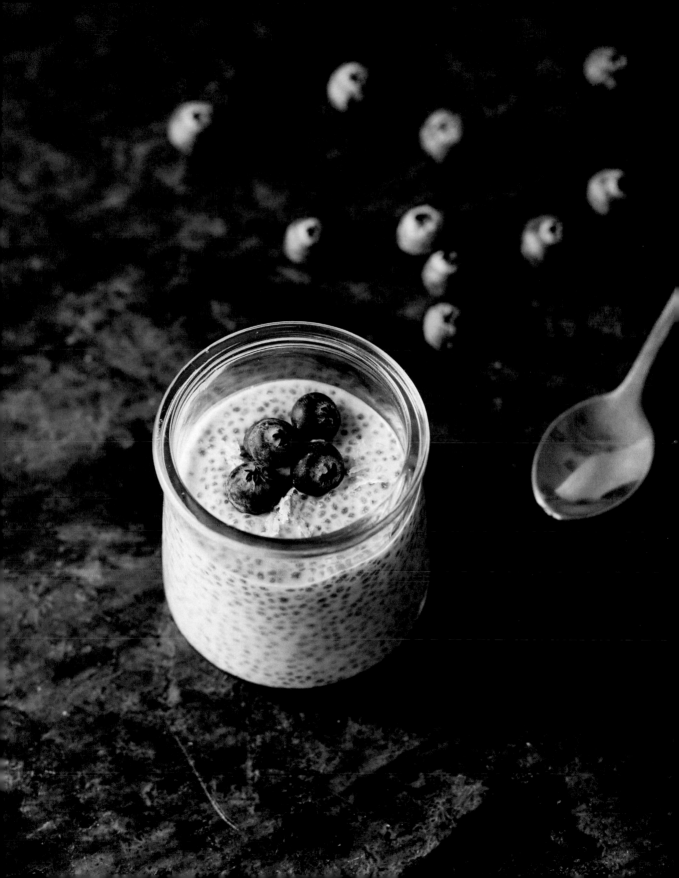

GRAWNOLA

SERVES 8; MAKES 4 CUPS
Prep and Cook Time: 30 minutes

3 cups old-fashioned rolled oats
¼ cup sunflower seeds
½ teaspoon coarsely ground Celtic salt
¼ cup raw honey
¼ cup almond butter (see Doctor's Note)
¼ cup flaxseeds
½ cup dark raisins (optional for Maintenance Phase)

We typically think of granola as something inherently healthy. Alas, that assumption is incorrect. Most store-bought granolas are usually just another way to consume processed sugars, chemicals, and other preservatives that heat you up instead of boosting your metabolism. Even granolas from health food stores often contain coconut sugar and refined coconut oil. To address this, we created a plant-based, healthy granola without refined sugar, added oils, or preservatives. You can also replace the almond butter with organic peanut butter; see Note.

1   Preheat the oven to 350° F. Line a large baking sheet with parchment paper.

2   In a large bowl, combine the oats, sunflower seeds, and salt.

3   In the bottom of a double boiler, bring approximately 2 inches of water to a gentle boil, taking care to leave a gap between the water and the bottom of the double boiler insert. Once it is boiling, reduce the heat to low. Add the honey and almond butter to the top of the double boiler and stir until the two combine into a warm and melted mixture, approximately 45 seconds. (If you don't own a double boiler, you can make one using a small saucepan and glass bowl that sits on top.)

4   Pour the honey and almond butter mixture over the

oat mixture, and stir to combine. Add the flaxseeds and stir again.

5   Spread the mixture evenly on the prepared baking sheet and bake for 18 to 20 minutes, or until golden brown and crunchy.

6   Remove the baking sheet from the oven and, if using, add the raisins to the mixture. Let cool and transfer to an airtight jar. This will keep well in the pantry for up to 2 weeks.

DOCTOR'S NOTE   When using nut butters, look for ones made with raw or dry roasted (unsalted) nuts.

NOTE   You can substitute ⅓ cup organic peanut butter for the almond butter; if so, increase the honey to ⅓ cup. Follow this recipe's instructions, except bake for 13 to 15 minutes.

Cinnamon Raisin
GRAWNOLA

SERVES 6

Prep and Cook Time: 25 minutes

---

3 cups old-fashioned rolled oats

2 teaspoons ground cinnamon

½ teaspoon coarsely ground
Celtic salt

¾ cup unsweetened applesauce

2 tablespoons raw honey

¼ cup unsweetened sunflower seed
butter

½ cup dark raisins

For those who would prefer a change of pace, or for those who can't have nuts, this nut-free "grAWnola" is made with applesauce, rolled oats, and sunflower-seed butter. It's a delicious cold-cereal substitute without preservatives or added sugars.

1 Preheat the oven to 350°F. Line a large baking sheet with parchment paper.

2 In a large bowl, combine the oats, cinnamon, and salt.

3 In a small bowl, combine the applesauce, honey, and sunflower seed butter. Stir well. Pour the wet mixture over the oat mixture, and stir to thoroughly combine.

4 Spread the mixture evenly on the lined baking sheet and bake for about 20 minutes, or until golden brown.

5 Remove from the oven and add the raisins to the baked mixture. Let cool. You can eat the granola right away or transfer it to an airtight jar for storage. It will keep well for up to 2 weeks.

HOT QUINOA BREAKFAST PORRIDGE
with Bosc Pear

SERVES 2
Prep and Cook Time: 20 minutes

½ cup uncooked white quinoa, rinsed and drained
1¼ cups nondairy milk, plus more (optional) for serving
¼ teaspoon ground cinnamon
1 tablespoon pure maple syrup
1 Bosc pear, cored and chopped
¼ cup chopped walnuts
¼ cup unsweetened coconut flakes

For a "heart-warming," gluten-free, whole-grain morning alternative to oatmeal, try this quinoa-based, dairy-free hot cereal. It's easy to make, tasty, and healthy.

1   Combine the quinoa and nondairy milk in a small saucepan. Bring to a boil, cover, and reduce the heat to low. Let it cook for 15 minutes.

2   Remove the saucepan from the heat and let sit, covered, for an additional 5 minutes.

3   Stir in the cinnamon and maple syrup.

4   Divide the quinoa between two bowls, and top each with half the chopped pear, walnuts, and coconut. Top off with more nondairy milk, if desired. Serve.

SNACKS, SPREADS, AND SIDES

H HEALING PHASE   M MAINTENANCE PHASE

Nut and Seed
POWER BAR

MAKES 10 BARS
Prep Time: 45 minutes

---

1 cup raw organic almonds
½ cup raw unsalted cashews
¼ cup chia seeds
3 ounces Deglet dates, pitted
   (about 12 dates)
8 ounces dried Turkish apricots
   (about 30 apricots)
3 tablespoons filtered water

For those who desire a nut-based bar that can give you a week's worth of healthy snacking, this tree-nut, chia-seed delight with dates and dried apricots hits the spot.

1   Line a 9 × 5-inch loaf pan with a piece of parchment paper so that the excess hangs over the longest sides and set aside (see Note). The parchment is not intended to keep the pan clean but rather makes transferring the bars out of the pan easy.

2   Combine all the ingredients in the bowl of a food processor. Pulse until the mixture gathers into a ball or mound but chunks remain, about 1 minute.

3   With damp hands, press the mixture into an even layer in the lined loaf pan. Refrigerate for at least 30 minutes to set.

4   To serve, lift the mixture out of the pan using the parchment paper as a vehicle and slice into 10 bars. Cover and store in the refrigerator for up to 1 week.

NOTE   If you don't have a loaf pan, you can use a small baking dish. Just remember that the size of the dish may change the thickness and/or quantity of the bars.

Puffed Kamut Sunflower Seed BUTTER BAR

MAKES 10 BARS
Prep Time: 45 minutes

12 ounces Deglet dates, pitted (about 50 dates)
½ cup unsweetened sunflower seed butter
1 teaspoon pure vanilla extract
2 tablespoons filtered water
⅛ teaspoon finely ground Celtic salt
1½ cups puffed Kamut cereal
½ cup sunflower seeds
½ cup unsweetened coconut flakes

Kamut is a wheat-based grain that is the bedrock of this nut-free bar.

1   Line a 9 × 5-inch loaf pan with parchment paper so that the excess hangs over the longest sides and set aside (see Note). The parchment is not intended to keep the pan clean but rather makes transferring the bars out of the pan easy.

2   In the bowl of a food processor, combine the dates, sunflower seed butter, vanilla, filtered water, and salt. Process until the mixture gathers into a ball or mound, about 2 minutes. Transfer to a large bowl. Pour in the Kamut, sunflower seeds, and coconut, and knead until thoroughly combined. With your hands, press the dough evenly into the lined loaf pan. Refrigerate for 30 minutes to set.

3   To serve, lift the mixture out of the pan using the parchment paper as a vehicle and slice into 10 bars. Cover and store in the refrigerator for up to 1 week.

NOTE   If you don't have a loaf pan, you can use a small baking dish. Just remember that the size of the dish may change the thickness and/or quantity of the bars.

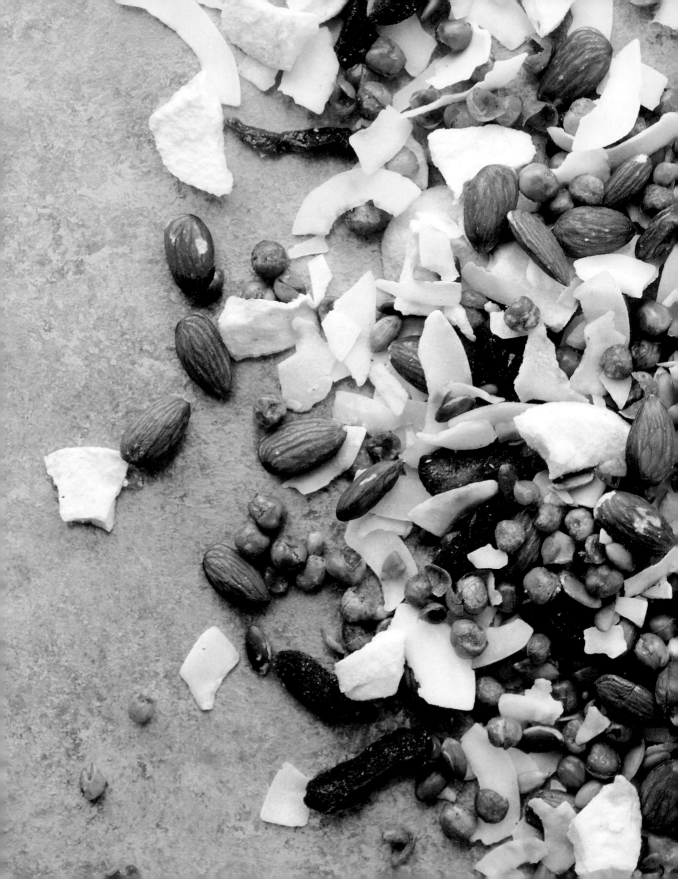

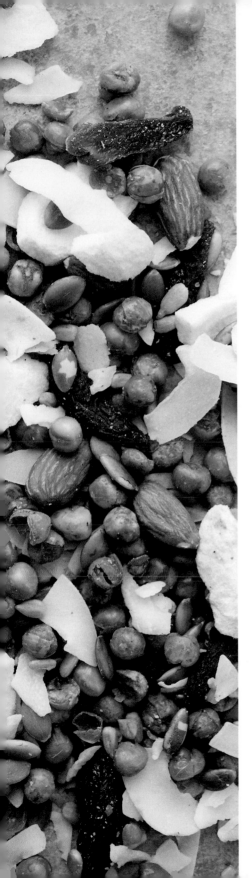

Texture and Color Riot
TRAIL MIX

**SERVES 6,
APPROXIMATELY 2 TABLESPOONS PER SERVING**
Prep and Cook Time: 10 minutes

This isn't your ordinary trail mix, loaded with salted pretzels, sugary granola, and other processed additives. This Acid Watcher version without inflammatory preservatives is chewy, crunchy, soft, and bursting with colors. If served in small portions, it's a satisfying and healthy hunger quencher. This recipe calls for dehydrated apples, which are made without additives and sold at most grocery stores.

⅓ cup raw organic almonds
2 tablespoons pepitas (pumpkin seeds)
1 tablespoon sunflower seeds
5 ounces dehydrated apples, crumbled
2 tablespoons unsweetened coconut flakes
8 to 10 dried Turkish apricots, cut into strips
2 tablespoons roasted peas

1   In a small nonstick pan, toast the almonds, pepitas, and sunflower seeds over medium heat for 2 to 5 minutes, until the nuts and seeds begin to release their aroma. Transfer them to a medium bowl. Add the apples, coconut, apricots, and peas, and mix thoroughly.

2   Serve in a bowl or divide into 2-tablespoon portions and store in an airtight container at room temperature for up to 5 days.

APPLE AND PEAR SAUCE

SERVES 2
Prep Time: 5 minutes

1 Bosc pear, cored and halved
1 Golden Delicious or Gala apple, cored and halved (see Doctor's Note)
⅛ cup filtered water

This delicious and easy-to-make apple-pear sauce is terrific as a snack on its own.

Combine all the ingredients in a blender and blend until smooth. Pour into two small bowls and enjoy immediately, or if you would like it cold, refrigerate for an hour in an airtight jar, then enjoy it.

DOCTOR'S NOTE When one purees Gala apples alone, the pH drops from 4.31 to below 4.0. To counteract this acidity, we added a Bosc pear, raising the pH and making the entire sauce more alkaline.

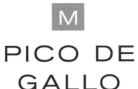

PICO DE GALLO

SERVES 2
Prep Time: 10 minutes

½ cup quartered grape tomatoes
1 tablespoon chopped fresh cilantro
¼ teaspoon finely ground Celtic salt
½ teaspoon lime zest

Acid Watchers tend to be wary of Mexican food; however, that is about to change. This pico de gallo salsa is Acid Watcher friendly and quick and easy to make. Fresh lime zest is used to replace the acidic lime juice.

Combine the tomatoes, cilantro, salt, and lime zest in a bowl and mix thoroughly with a spoon. Serve with the Acid Watcher Cracker (page 93), Baked Corn Tortilla Chips (page 92), Huevos Rancheros (page 57), or straight from the spoon. You can store the Pico de Gallo in an airtight container in the refrigerator for 24 hours.

REAL! GUACAMOLE

SERVES 2
Prep Time: 10 minutes

2 medium to large ripe Hass
   avocados, peeled and pitted
1 tablespoon fresh lime juice
   (see Doctor's Note)
½ teaspoon coarsely ground
   Celtic salt
⅓ cup quartered grape tomatoes
¼ cup chopped fresh cilantro
Baked Corn Tortilla Chips
   (page 92), for serving
   (optional)
Sliced jicama, celery, and/or carrots,
   for serving (optional)

You would be hard-pressed to find an Acid Watcher who doesn't desperately miss regular old guacamole! The fresh cilantro, tomato, and lime juice in this easy-to-make guacamole fully compensates for the loss of raw onion while saving all of us that dreaded dragon breath and an upset stomach. We all agree that it's just such a relief to have real guac back—and bonus points for guac that actually stays green!

1   Scoop out the flesh of the avocados and place it in a bowl. Add the lime juice and salt to the bowl and mash the mixture with a fork until the lime juice has been absorbed by the avocado.

2   Add the quartered tomatoes and chopped cilantro and stir to combine.

3   Enjoy with tortilla chips and/or sliced jicama, celery, and carrots, if desired.

DOCTOR'S NOTE   The lime's acidity is neutralized by the avocado's alkalinity.

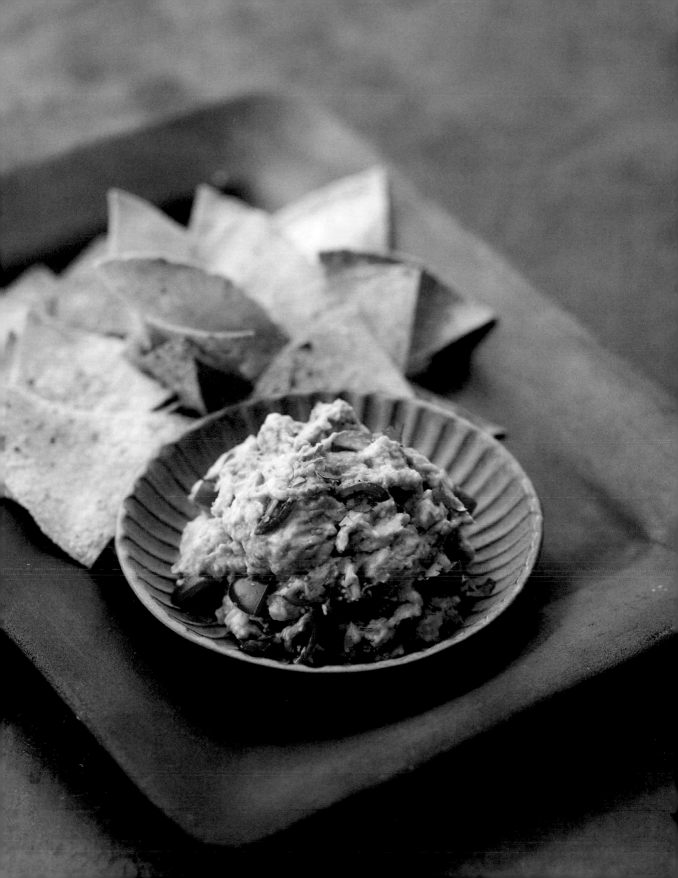

CHOPPED "LIVER"

SERVES 4
Prep and Cook Time: 20 minutes

---

1 cup chopped onion
  (1 medium onion)
1 teaspoon olive oil
1 cup raw walnut halves
2 large hard-boiled eggs
10 ounces sweet peas, fresh or
  thawed frozen
½ teaspoon coarsely ground
  Celtic salt

This meat-free rendition combines peas, hard-boiled eggs, sautéed onion, and walnuts to create a delicious, healthy snack that is full of fiber. It's delicious by itself or on the Acid Watcher Cracker (page 93) or Baked Corn Tortilla Chips (page 92).

1   In a medium skillet over medium heat, sauté the onions in the oil for 7 to 8 minutes, until tender and slightly golden brown. Remove from the heat and let cool.

2   In the bowl of a food processor, pulse the walnuts until crushed, about 30 seconds. Add the hard-boiled egg, onions, peas, and salt to the crushed walnuts and puree the mixture until smooth, scraping down the sides of the bowl as necessary. Transfer the mixture to a bowl and serve.

REAL HUMMUS

SERVES 2

Prep Time: 10 minutes

---

1 (15-ounce) can organic chickpeas

¼ cup tahini

1 tablespoon olive oil

¼ to ½ teaspoon coarsely ground Celtic salt

3 tablespoons fresh lemon juice (see Doctor's Note)

2 tablespoons aquafaba

1 teaspoon za'atar

Chopped fresh parsley, for garnish

Sliced carrots, celery, and/or the Acid Watcher Cracker (page 93), for serving (optional)

Store-bought hummus often contains acids, preservatives, raw garlic, and/or onion—all things that are hazardous to an Acid Watcher. In this Maintenance Phase–appropriate hummus, the Middle Eastern spice *za'atar*, which contains herbs such as ground dried thyme, oregano, marjoram, sesame seeds, and sumac, is added and provides a woodsy, citrusy flavor to the dish without having to use large quantities of fresh lemon.

Acid Watchers are also used to staying clear of canned and jarred foods, or at least draining and rinsing all foods found in a can as they typically contain added acid and preservatives. Meet the exception: the canned chickpea. The liquid found in the can of chickpeas—called *aquafaba*—is a miracle product for the Acid Watcher. Not only does it thin out this hummus but—as opposed to alkaline water—it also raises the pH of the mixture.

1 Drain but do not rinse the chickpeas, and reserve the aquafaba (liquid) from the can.

2 Combine the drained chickpeas, tahini, olive oil, salt, lemon juice, and aquafaba in the bowl of a food processor. Pulse until creamy and well combined, scraping down the sides of the bowl as necessary.

3 Transfer the hummus to a bowl and top with the za'atar and parsley. Serve immediately with sliced carrots, celery, and/or crackers. Cover and store leftovers in the refrigerator for up to a week.

DOCTOR'S NOTE The lemon's acidity is neutralized by the alkalinity of the chickpeas, aquafaba, and tahini.

MAGRA'S BABA
(*Baba Ghanouj*)

SERVES 2
Prep and Cook Time: 1 hour

1 medium eggplant, sliced crosswise
   into ¼-inch rounds (see Doctor's
   Note)
¾ teaspoon finely ground Celtic salt,
   plus more as needed
1 cup chopped onion
   (1 medium onion)
1 tablespoon olive oil, plus more for
   the eggplant
2 large hard-boiled eggs

Magra is an affectionate nickname our children have for their grandmother, who not only has an unusual nickname but also makes an unusually tasty and healthy eggplant-based spread.

1   Preheat the broiler and position a rack 4 to 6 inches from the broiler. Line a large baking sheet with aluminum foil and set it aside.

2   Sprinkle the eggplant rounds lightly with salt on both sides and place them in a colander for 10 minutes to draw out the excess moisture.

3   While the eggplant is resting, in a medium skillet over medium heat, sauté the onions in the olive oil for 7 to 8 minutes, until tender and slightly golden brown. Remove from the heat and let cool.

4   When you return to your eggplant, you should observe little droplets of water on each round. Pat each round dry with paper towels and lay them flat on your lined baking sheet. Using a pastry brush, lightly brush both sides of the eggplant with the olive oil. Broil for about 5 minutes, or until golden brown. Turn the eggplant and broil the other sides for about another 5 minutes, or until golden brown.

5   Remove the baking sheet from the oven and wrap the eggplant slices in the aluminum foil to create a sealed pouch. Let the eggplant rest in the pouch, *outside the oven,* for 5 minutes. Then carefully open the packet and let the eggplant cool.

6   In the bowl of a food processor, combine the hard-boiled eggs, cooked onion, eggplant, and salt, and pulse for 1 minute, scraping down the sides of the bowl to incorporate the ingredients as necessary. The final mixture should retain some texture.

7   Transfer the mixture to a bowl, season with salt to taste, and serve immediately, or refrigerate, covered, and enjoy chilled within 24 hours.

DOCTOR'S NOTE   Typically, baba ghanouj recipes call for removing the eggplant skin, while the Acid Watcher version leaves the eggplant skin on. There are two reasons we keep the eggplant skin. One is the greater amount of fiber that is found in the skin. The other is a phytonutrient (natural chemical found in plants) found in eggplant skin called *nasunin*. Nasunin is a potent antioxidant that protects cell membranes from damage, in particular fat cells in the brain, hence one of the reasons eggplant is often referred to as "brain food."

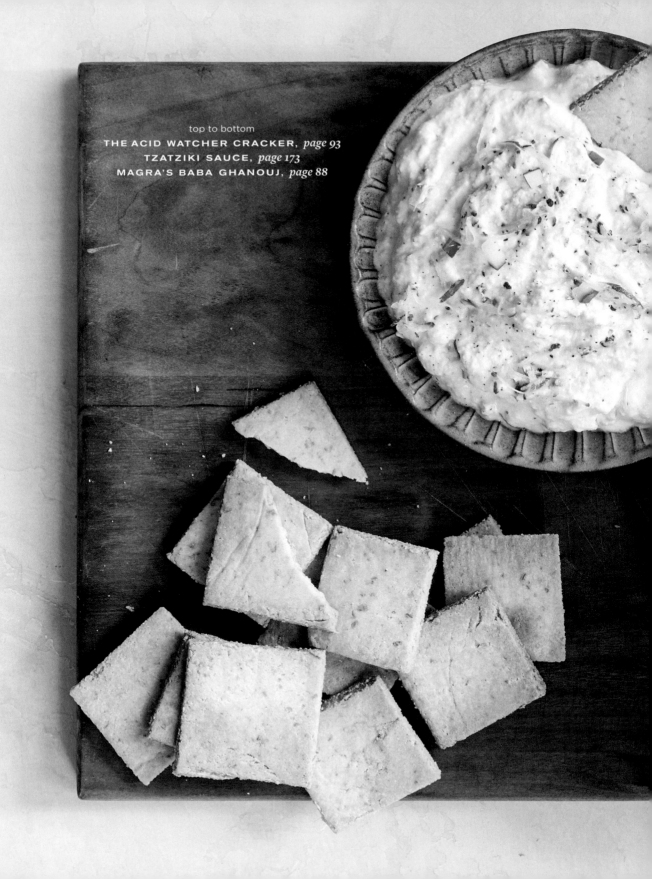

top to bottom
THE ACID WATCHER CRACKER, *page 93*
TZATZIKI SAUCE, *page 173*
MAGRA'S BABA GHANOUJ, *page 88*

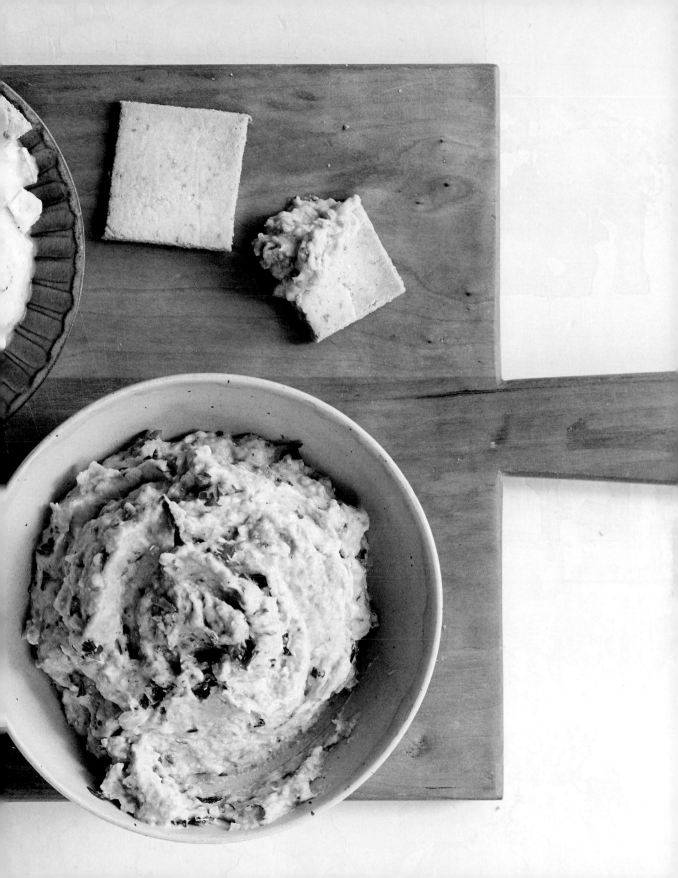

Baked Corn
TORTILLA CHIPS

MAKES 24 CHIPS
Prep and Cook Time: 25 minutes

---

4 corn tortillas, preferably Trader
  Joe's Corn Tortillas or Ezekiel 4:9
  Sprouted Corn Tortillas
1 tablespoon olive oil
Coarsely ground Celtic salt to taste
Real! Guacamole (page 84) and/or
  Pico de Gallo (page 83), for serving
  (optional)

Continuing with the "make this, don't buy that" anti-inflammatory food ethos of the Acid Watcher Diet, these homemade "corn chips" use readily available preservative-free corn tortillas transformed into healthy chips for dips, sauces, and salads.

1   Preheat the oven to 400°F and line a large baking sheet with parchment paper.

2   Using a pastry brush, lightly coat one side of each tortilla with olive oil. Cut each tortilla into 6 equal wedges and place them, oil side up, on the baking sheet. Sprinkle with Celtic salt and bake for 15 to 20 minutes, until golden brown and crispy.

3   Serve with guacamole and/or pico de gallo, if desired. Store leftovers in an airtight container in a cool dry pantry for 2 to 3 days.

The Acid Watcher
CRACKER

**MAKES ABOUT FIFTY 1½-INCH
SQUARE CRACKERS**
Prep and Cook Time: 25 minutes

1 large egg
1½ cups almond flour
1 tablespoon wheat bran
½ teaspoon finely ground Celtic salt

One of the goals of this cookbook is to provide healthy substitutes for the salty, sugary, and fatty snacks that permeate our diets. These crackers have the mouthfeel and crunch of the snacks we are trying to move away from, while still providing a healthy alternative. This cracker is a wonderful accompaniment to the many spreads in this book.

1   Preheat the oven to 350°F.

2   In a large bowl, whisk the egg until smooth. Add the almond flour, wheat bran, and salt. Mix with your hands until it forms a homogeneous dough.

3   Place the dough between two pieces of parchment paper and roll it out until it is ¹⁄₁₆ inch thick. Then remove the top piece of parchment paper.

4   Transfer the bottom piece of parchment paper with the rolled-out dough onto a baking sheet. With a knife or a pizza cutter, cut the dough into 1½-inch squares and bake for 12 to 15 minutes, until evenly golden brown. Remove from the oven and let cool for 5 minutes, then serve. Leftovers may be stored in an airtight container in a cool dry pantry for 3 to 5 days.

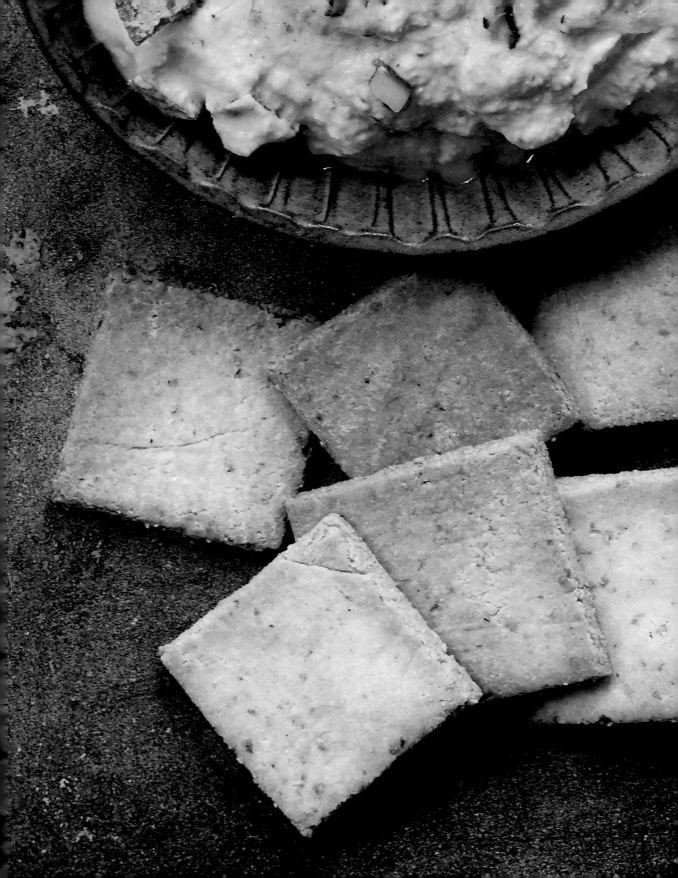

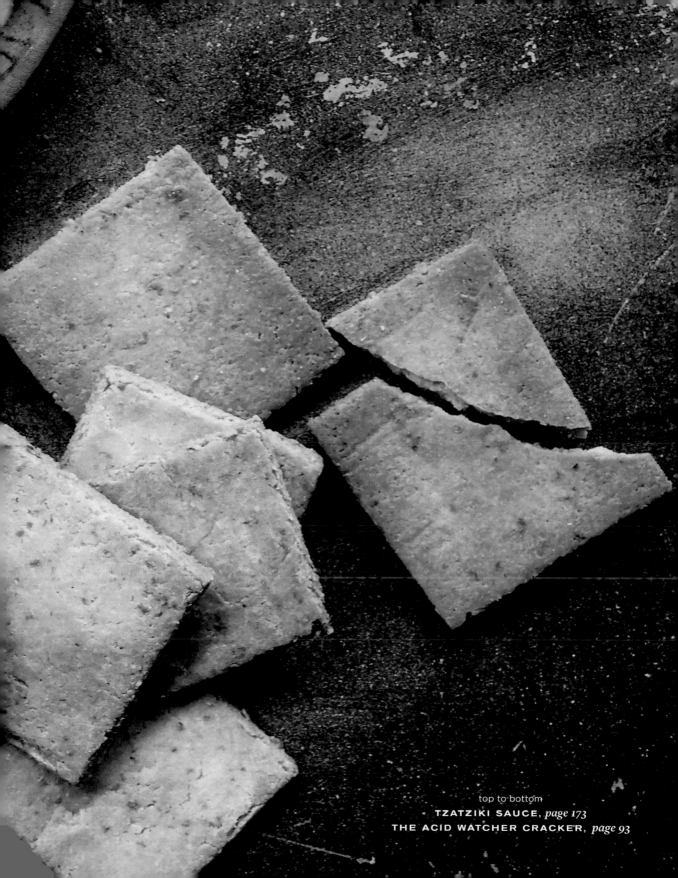

top to bottom
TZATZIKI SAUCE, *page 173*
THE ACID WATCHER CRACKER, *page 93*

BAKED CARROTS

SERVES 2
Prep and Cook Time: 1¼ hours

4 large carrots
Coarsely ground Celtic salt

This simple, delicious, sweet, and savory carrot side dish will win over anyone who doesn't like veggies.

1   Preheat the oven to 400°F.

2   Peel the carrots, sprinkle with salt, wrap in foil, and place the packet on a baking sheet. Bake for about 1 hour, or until the carrots are tender when pierced with a fork.

3   Remove the carrots from the oven, remove the foil, and serve immediately.

MUSHROOM DRESSING

SERVES 4

Prep and Cook Time: 20 minutes

1 tablespoon coconut oil

3 cups mixed chopped mushrooms (shiitake, white button, oyster)

½ cup chopped Gala apple

½ cup chopped onion

1 clove fresh garlic, minced (optional)

3 to 4 tablespoons AW Vegetable Broth (page 112)

1 tablespoon chopped fresh parsley

½ tablespoon chopped fresh rosemary

½ teaspoon chopped fresh thyme

¼ teaspoon coarsely ground Celtic salt

This grain-free side dish is a delicious accompaniment to a casual weeknight dinner or to a traditional Thanksgiving meal.

1   In a large skillet over high heat, melt the coconut oil; add the chopped mushrooms, apple, onions, and garlic (if using). Sauté for 8 to 10 minutes, stirring occasionally, until *both* the mixture sticks to the bottom of the skillet and browning occurs on the bottom of the skillet.

2   Add the vegetable broth, a tablespoon at a time, using the broth to deglaze the bottom of the skillet. Remove the skillet from the heat.

3   Stir in the parsley, rosemary, thyme, and salt, and transfer to a serving bowl and serve immediately.

TZATZIKI SAUCE, *page 173*

ZUCCHINI FRIES

SERVES 2

Prep and Cook Time: 40 minutes

2 medium zucchini
3 large eggs
2 cups puffed brown rice cereal
½ teaspoon finely ground Celtic salt

Who doesn't like the shoestring zucchini fries that seem to work their way into your meal, masquerading as a "health food" while you're asking someone for more paper towels to soak up the grease? Here comes the Acid Watcher version of zucchini fries—baked, not fried—to the rescue!

1   Preheat the oven to 425°F. Place a wire cooling rack on a baking sheet and set it aside.

2   Cut the ends off each zucchini. Cut the zucchini lengthwise into ¼-inch-thick slices, then cut each slice into ¼-inch sticks and set aside.

3   Beat the eggs in a wide shallow bowl.

4   In the bowl of a food processor, grind the puffed rice for 10 to 15 seconds, just until it resembles breadcrumbs. Transfer the rice to another wide shallow bowl. Stir in the salt.

5   Gently dip the zucchini sticks into the egg mixture to coat evenly, letting the excess drip back into the bowl. Then coat each stick with the ground rice.

6   Arrange all of the breaded zucchini fries on the cooling rack fitted in the baking sheet. Bake for 15 to 20 minutes, until golden brown and crispy. Serve immediately.

SWEET POTATO MASH

SERVES 2

Prep and Cook Time: 40 minutes

---

2 medium sweet potatoes, peeled
½ tablespoon pure maple syrup
¼ teaspoon ground cinnamon
1 tablespoon almond milk
Coarsely ground Celtic salt

Sweet potatoes rule. They're scrumptious and full of antioxidants, vitamin A, and fiber.

1   Bring a medium saucepan of water to a boil.

2   Meanwhile, cut each peeled sweet potato into 4 to 6 chunks. Add the sweet potatoes to the boiling water and cook for 20 to 30 minutes, until tender. Drain the sweet potatoes well and transfer them to a blender. Add the maple syrup, cinnamon, and almond milk to the blender and blend until smooth.

3   Transfer the mixture to a bowl and season to taste with salt. Serve immediately.

GREEN BEANS "ALMONDINE"

SERVES 2
Prep and Cook Time: 15 minutes

½ pound green beans, ends trimmed
1 tablespoon olive oil
¼ cup raw sliced almonds
½ teaspoon finely ground Celtic salt

Fun with veggies continues in this Acid Watcher–friendly iteration of green beans amandine. Toasting the almonds brings a rich, earthy flavor to the entire dish.

1   Bring a large pot of water to a boil over high heat; add the green beans. Boil the green beans for 2 minutes, then drain and set aside to cool.

2   In a large frying pan over medium heat, combine the olive oil and almonds. Slowly toast the almonds, stirring occasionally until golden brown, 5 to 6 minutes. Add the green beans and salt, and toss to coat completely. Serve immediately.

ARTICHOKES
with Garlic Aioli

SERVES 2
Prep and Cook Time: 45 minutes

2 dried bay leaves
¼ teaspoon finely ground Celtic salt
2 artichokes
Garlic Aioli (page 171)

Raw cashews are the "secret sauce" in this otherwise acidic recipe. This restaurant-style artichoke appetizer or side dish will impress your guests. What puts this over the top is a dairy-free, nutrient-rich, cooked-garlic aioli that tastes just like the dairy version!

1   Using a pot large enough to hold your artichokes, fill it halfway with water. Add the bay leaves and salt to the pot. Cover with a tight-fitting lid and bring the water to a boil.

2   While your water is working its way to a boil, rinse the artichokes and, using a serrated bread knife, slice off the bottom stems flush with the base so that they stand level.

3   Place the artichokes, stem end down, in the boiling water and reduce the heat to a simmer. Cover with a tight-fitting lid and simmer for 35 to 40 minutes, until the base of each artichoke can easily be pierced with a knife.

4   Drain the artichokes in a colander with the pointed top end facing downward. Once the artichokes have expelled their water, place each in a serving dish, right side up, and serve immediately with the garlic aioli. Alternatively, the artichokes can be refrigerated and served cold with the garlic aioli.

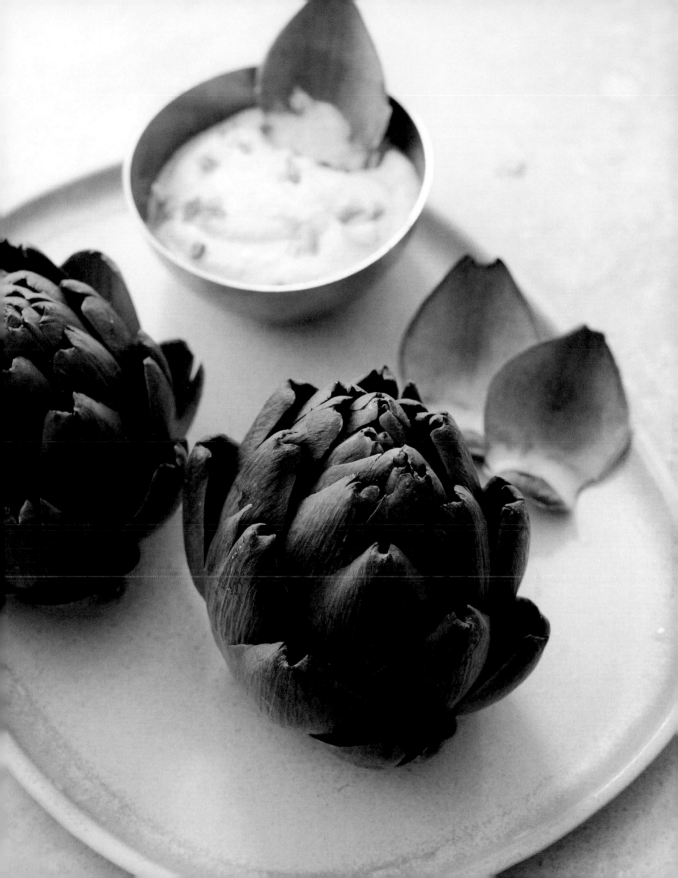

Cauliflower
"FRIED" RICE

SERVES 2

Prep and Cook Time: 20 minutes

2½ teaspoons olive oil

2 large eggs, whisked

⅓ cup chopped onion

3 cups riced cauliflower,
  store-bought or homemade
  (see Note)

⅓ cup sweet peas, fresh or thawed
  frozen

1 tablespoon soy sauce

Coarsely ground Celtic salt

For those of you who look longingly at a fried rice dish but do not want to deal with the inflammatory oils and white rice, now there is a healthy veggie-based alternative. This extremely versatile side dish is great with Grilled Salmon with Crispy Skin (page 137) or Ed's Sunday Night Whole Roast Chicken (page 160).

1   Warm ½ teaspoon of the olive oil in a large nonstick pan over medium-high heat. Once the oil is warm, add the eggs and scramble them as desired. Transfer the eggs to a small bowl and set them aside. Clean the pan with a paper towel.

2   Add 1 teaspoon of the olive oil to the cleaned pan over medium-high heat. Add the onions and cook until golden brown.

3   Quickly add the cauliflower, peas, remaining 1 teaspoon olive oil, and soy sauce, and sauté for about 3 minutes, stirring continuously. Return the scrambled eggs to the pan and sauté everything for another minute.

4   Divide the dish between two plates, sprinkle with salt to taste, and serve.

NOTE   To prepare riced cauliflower, remove the core and leaves of 2 large heads of cauliflower, and roughly chop the florets. Add the cauliflower to the bowl of a food processor in batches—fill it about halfway each time. Pulse slowly until the cauliflower is coarsely ground and resembles the size and texture of rice.

STEAMED ASPARAGUS
with Shaved Parmesan

SERVES 2
Prep and Cook Time: 10 minutes

¼ teaspoon finely ground Celtic salt
12 asparagus spears
1 to 2 ounces shaved Parmesan cheese

Like most vegetables, asparagus is relatively alkaline (around pH 6). Further, each cup of asparagus contains about 4 grams of fiber plus numerous vitamins and minerals, making it an ideal Healing Phase side.

1 In a large pot that will hold a steamer basket, pour approximately 1 inch of water (the water should go up to the bottom of the steamer basket but not over the asparagus). Add the salt and bring the water to a boil over high heat.

2 While the water comes to a boil, clean and trim the bottom 2 inches of each asparagus spear. Place the asparagus in the steamer basket.

3 Once the water is boiling, lower the steamer basket with the asparagus into the pot and cover with a tight-fitting lid. Keep the water boiling.

4 Steam the asparagus for 5 to 7 minutes, until the spears are tender. Transfer the asparagus to two plates, top with the shaved Parmesan, and serve.

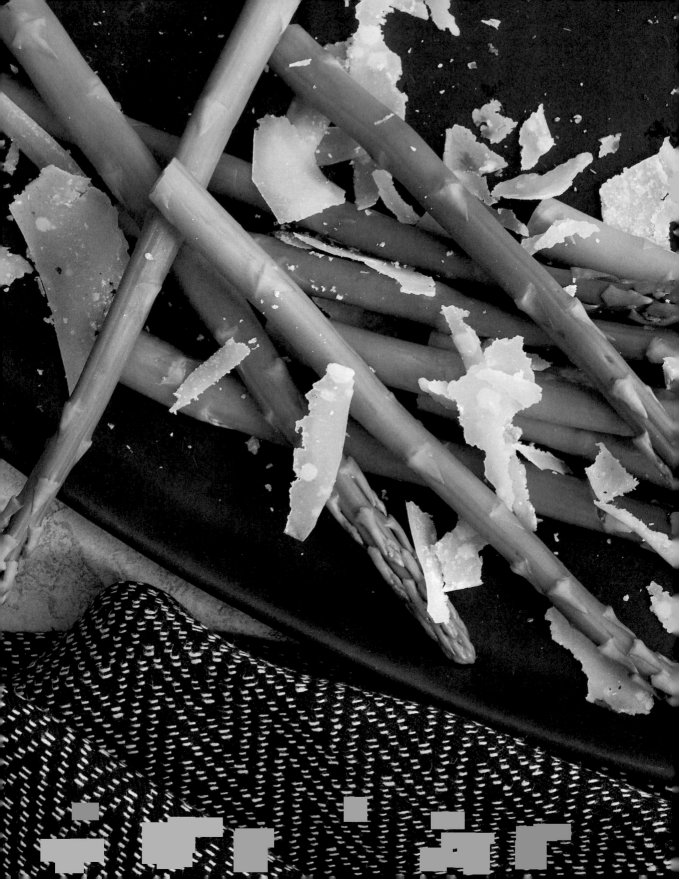

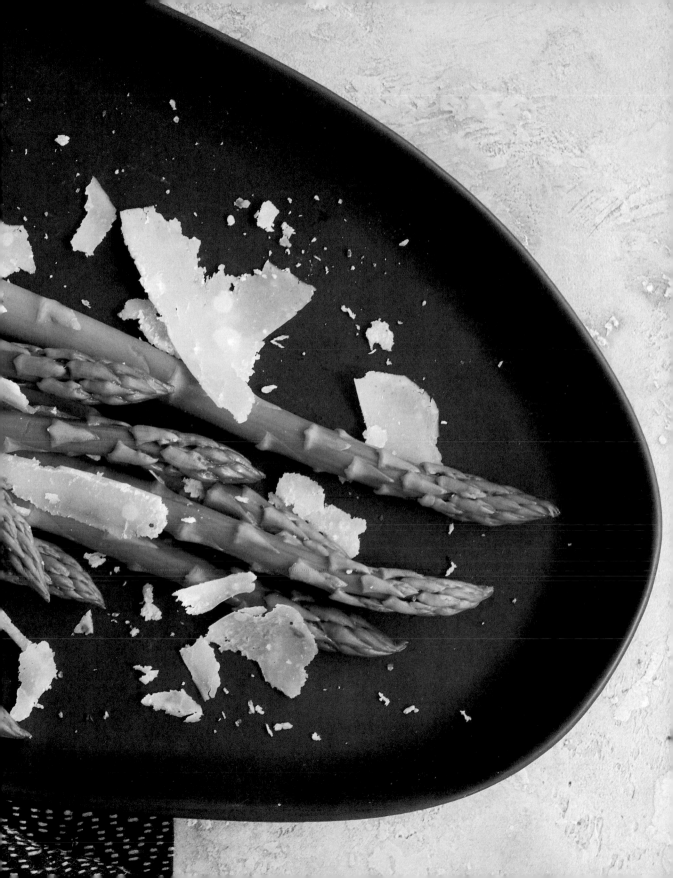

Celtic-Salted

KALE CHIPS

SERVES 2

Prep and Cook Time: 20 minutes

This easy-to-make savory, salty, and crunchy side dish is a healthy (baked, not fried) accompaniment to game-day finger food.

2 bunches curly kale, stemmed and coarsely chopped
2 tablespoons olive oil
½ teaspoon coarsely ground Celtic salt

1   Preheat the oven to 350°F. Line a large baking sheet with parchment paper and set it aside.

2   In a large bowl, toss the kale with the olive oil and salt. Spread the kale evenly, in a single layer on the lined baking sheet, and bake for approximately 15 minutes, until crispy but not burnt, then remove from the oven.

3   Serve the kale chips warm or let cool for snacking during halftime.

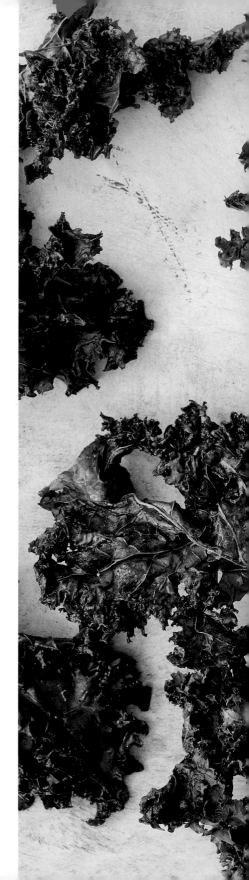

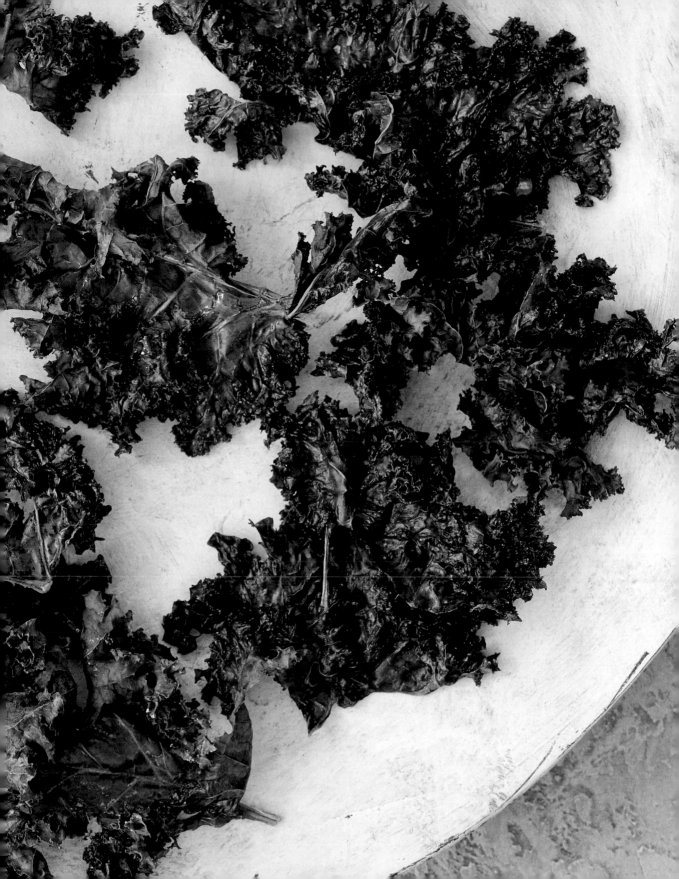

SOUPS AND SALADS

H HEALING PHASE   M MAINTENANCE PHASE

AW VEGETABLE BROTH

MAKES APPROXIMATELY 6 CUPS
Prep and Cook Time: 1½ hours

½ teaspoon olive oil
7 celery stalks, coarsely chopped
5 carrots, cleaned and coarsely
    chopped (peeling optional)
2 parsnips, cleaned and coarsely
    chopped (peeling optional)
2 teaspoons finely ground Celtic salt
1 bay leaf
1 bunch fresh parsley
1 bunch fresh dill

This alkaline vegetable broth, without onion or garlic, is thus Acid Watcher friendly during the Healing Phase and forms the basis of various dishes in this cookbook.

1   Heat the oil in a large pot over medium heat. Add the celery, carrots, parsnips, and ½ teaspoon of the salt, and sauté over medium high heat until fragrant and lightly golden, about 10 minutes. Pour in 8 cups of water, 1 teaspoon salt, and the bay leaf. Bring to a boil, cover partially with a lid, then reduce the heat to a simmer. Cook for 45 minutes. Add the parsley and dill, and cook for another 15 minutes.

2   Strain the broth through a fine sieve and season with the remaining ½ teaspoon salt. Use the refrigerated broth within 5 days, or freeze in airtight containers for up to 2 months.

MISO SOUP

SERVES 2

Prep and Cook Time: 20 minutes

1 tablespoon wakame
6 tablespoons plain white miso
  (not sweet white miso)
¼ (14-ounce) block tofu (soft or firm
  will work), cut into small cubes

Welcome to wakame, an edible seaweed generally available from many food retailers. It is usually sold dried and is a powerful natural anti-inflammatory agent that bolsters the health benefits of traditional miso soup.

1   In a small bowl, cover the wakame with water by about 1 inch. Set it aside.

2   In a medium saucepan, bring 5 cups of water to a boil over high heat. Turn off the heat and whisk in the miso until it dissolves almost entirely. Strain the miso broth through a fine-mesh sieve into a large bowl. Drain and rinse the wakame. Stir the wakame and tofu into the soup and serve immediately.

LENTIL SOUP

SERVES 2
Prep and Cook Time: 1 hour

---

1 tablespoon olive oil

1 large carrot, peeled and chopped (about ¾ cup)

3 celery stalks, chopped (about ¾ cup)

1½ teaspoons finely ground Celtic salt

6 cups AW Vegetable Broth (page 112)

¾ cup green lentils, rinsed and drained

Chopped fresh parsley, for garnish

Lentils and carrots and celery, oh my! Unlike typical lentil soup that includes ingredients like onion, garlic, and tomato, which can cause bloating and inflammation, this version combines the legumes with our basic vegetable broth and simple veggies to create a robust, delectable meal.

1   Warm a large pot over medium-high heat. Add the olive oil, carrot, celery, and salt, and sauté for about 3 minutes, until softened.

2   Pour in the broth and stir in the lentils. Bring the mixture to a boil, then reduce the heat and simmer, partially covered, for about 45 minutes, until the lentils are tender.

3   Ladle the soup into two bowls, garnish with parsley, and serve.

Plant-Based
CHILI

SERVES 2
Prep and Cook Time: 40 minutes

---

2 teaspoons olive oil

½ (8-ounce) block tempeh, crumbled

½ teaspoon finely ground Celtic salt

2 cups chopped portobello mushrooms (about 2 medium)

1 teaspoon ground cumin

1 teaspoon sweet paprika

2 cups chopped fresh tomatoes with their juices

2 cups AW Vegetable Broth (page 112), plus more (optional) as needed

1 cup black beans, rinsed and drained (about half of a 15-ounce can)

½ cup fresh or frozen corn kernels

1 tablespoon lime zest

2 tablespoons chopped fresh cilantro

1 avocado, peeled, pitted, and chopped

Cooked brown rice, for serving (optional)

The debate about what makes chili "chili" is particularly contentious, with a spectrum of ingredients in play, starting with no beans ever to beans always. Further complicating this passionate discussion is meat or no meat, what types of chiles, and which spices should be used. As one can imagine, the International Chili Society would roll over in their proverbial kitchen with the Acid Watcher rendition. But this plant-based version is savory and tasty, without meat, chile peppers, chili powder, or onions. Instead, using tempeh, mushrooms, tomatoes, black beans, lime zest, and a variety of cooked spices, our meatless chili is born.

1   In a large pot over medium-high heat, warm the olive oil. Add the tempeh and ¼ teaspoon of the salt, and sauté for about 2 minutes, until lightly browned. Add the portobello mushrooms and the remaining ¼ teaspoon salt. Cook 5 minutes longer, stirring occasionally, and add 2 tablespoons of water, the cumin, and paprika. Stir and cook for 1 more minute.

2   Add the chopped tomatoes and sauté for 2 to 3 minutes, stirring occasionally, until the tomatoes start to break down. Add the vegetable broth, reduce the heat to medium, and simmer for about 10 minutes, until slightly thickened. Stir in the black beans, corn kernels, and lime zest, and simmer for an additional 3 minutes. If the chili becomes too thick, add an additional splash of vegetable broth or water.

3   Divide the chili into two bowls and top each with the cilantro and chopped avocado. Serve with brown rice, if desired.

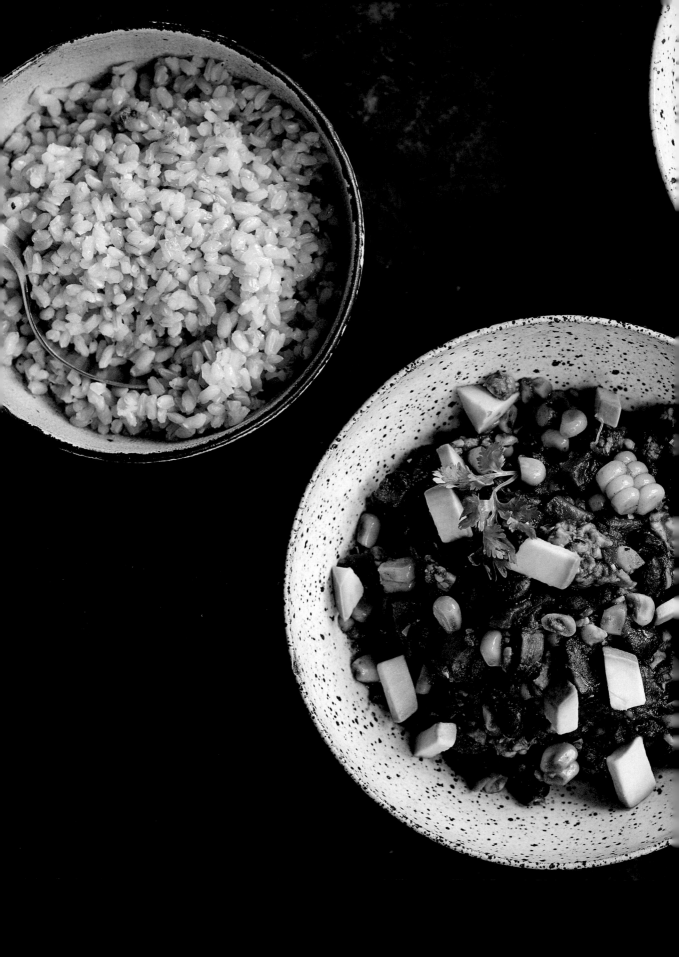

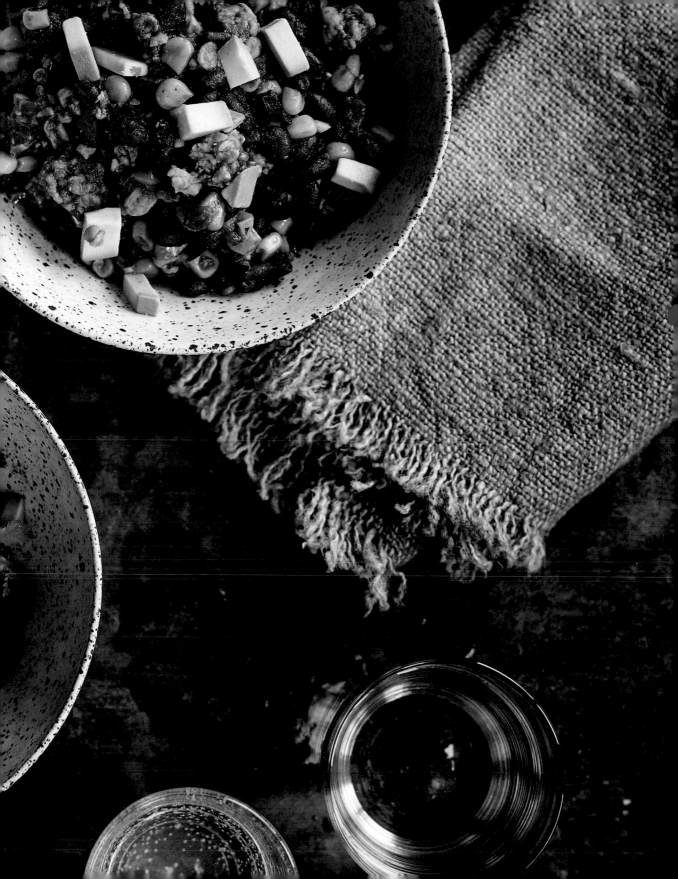

TOMATO BASIL SOUP

SERVES 2

Prep and Cook Time: 1¼ hours

1 pound plum tomatoes, halved
   lengthwise
2 carrots, peeled and coarsely
   chopped (approximately 1 cup
   chopped)
1 tablespoon olive oil
1½ teaspoons finely ground
   Celtic salt
1¼ cups AW Vegetable Broth
   (page 112)
5 fresh large basil leaves

This isn't the twilight zone. This is the Acid Watcher zone, where properly prepared tomatoes—that is, neutralized with carrots and vegetable broth—are used to create a Maintenance Phase soup.

1   Preheat the oven to 400°F. In a large bowl, toss the tomatoes and carrots with the olive oil and salt. Spread the mixture in an even layer on a baking sheet, and roast on the middle rack of the oven for 45 minutes, stirring halfway through, until the carrots and tomatoes are soft, juicy, and caramelized.

2   Transfer the roasted tomatoes and carrots and the vegetable broth to a blender and puree on high until smooth, about 1 minute. Add the basil leaves and pulse a few times, until they are coarsely chopped and speckle the soup. To serve, transfer the mixture to a saucepan and heat just until warmed through. Store in the refrigerator for up to 5 days or in the freezer for up to 1 month.

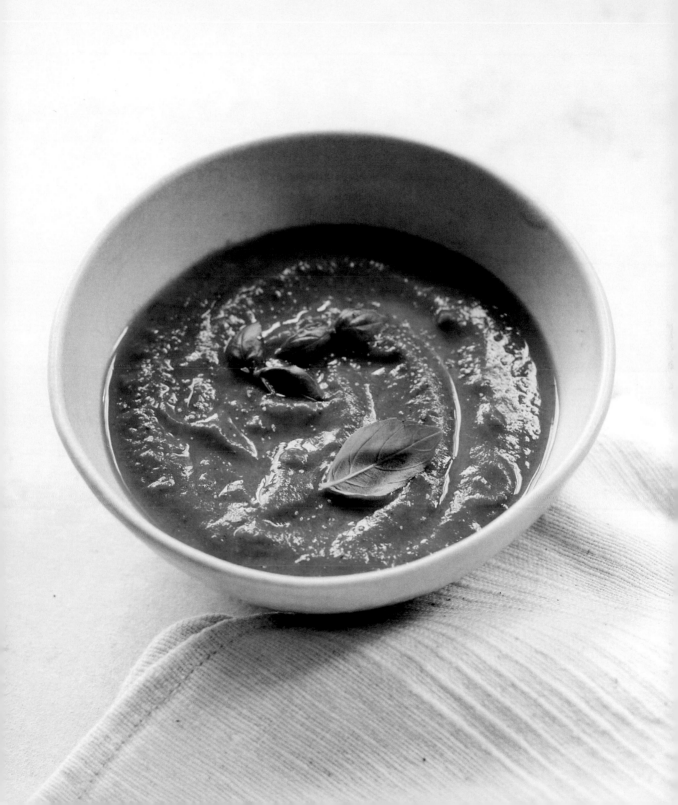

Fresh Pea
VICHYSSOISE

SERVES 6 TO 8

Prep and Cook Time: 1¼ hours,
plus 2 to 4 hours for chilling

---

2 tablespoons olive oil

1 leek, white and light green parts
only, cleaned and chopped

1 fennel bulb, cored, outer fibrous
leaves removed, coarsely chopped

4 ounces rutabaga, peeled and
chopped

2 ounces celery root, peeled and
chopped

2 celery stalks, chopped

Leaves of 2 fresh rosemary sprigs,
chopped

½ cup chopped fresh parsley leaves

2 teaspoons coarsely ground Celtic
salt

1 teaspoon herbes de Provence

1½ cups sweet peas, fresh or thawed
frozen

2 fresh bay leaves, or 1 dried

6 cups water

1 cup soy milk

The classic vichyssoise is a cold leek and potato soup flavored with butter, cream, chives, and herbs. Although the soup is considered a native of France's Provençal coast, it is actually American in origin. To make this summertime delight Acid Watcher–friendly, we've replaced the starchy potato with root vegetables and chives with the aromatic fennel. Instead of butter, we use olive oil, and soy milk replaces heavy cream. You'll get the unmistakable aroma of France with fresh rosemary and herbes de Provence. (If you can't find herbes de Provence in your grocery store, substitute dried thyme and culinary lavender.) This soup tastes best when it is silky smooth, so if you have a food mill, put it to use here; otherwise, use the immersion or regular blender to get the thinnest, smoothest consistency possible.

1   In a heavy-bottomed pot, preferably a Dutch oven, heat the olive oil over medium-high heat. Add the leek, fennel, rutabaga, celery root, celery, rosemary, parsley, salt, and herbes de Provence. Sauté, stirring frequently, for 12 to 15 minutes, until the root vegetables begin to soften and release their aroma. Add splashes of water, if necessary, to prevent them from sticking or burning.

2   Raise the temperature to high. Add the peas, bay leaves, and water, and bring the mixture to a boil. Reduce the temperature to low and simmer, partially

covered, for 45 minutes, stirring occasionally to prevent clumping. Skim the surface, if necessary. Remove from the heat and let the soup cool to room temperature.

3   Puree the cooled soup with a blender until smooth and whisk in the soy milk. For optimal results, run half the pureed soup through a food mill, if you have one, and return it to the pot. Cover and chill for 2 to 4 hours before serving.

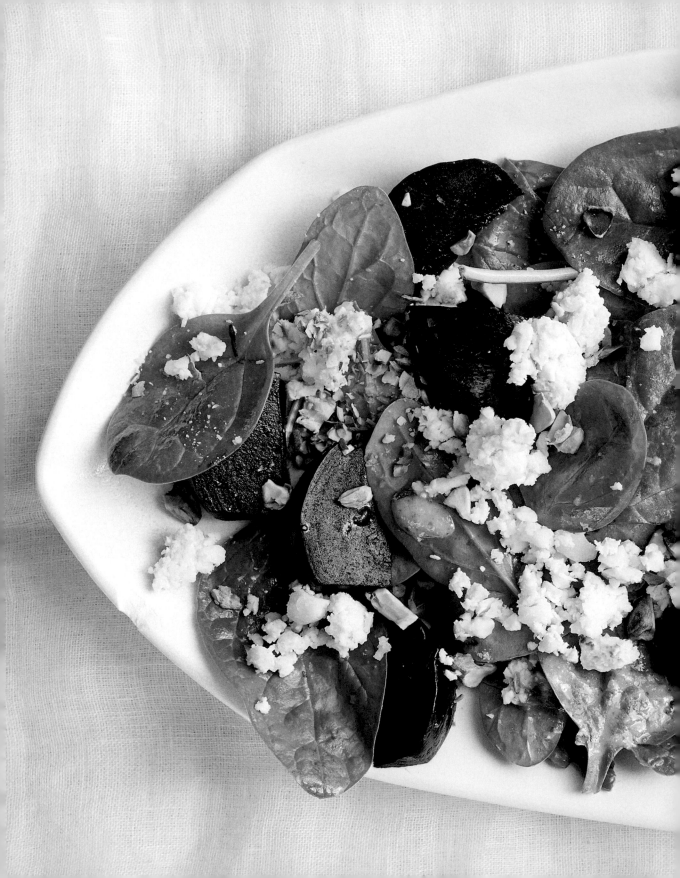

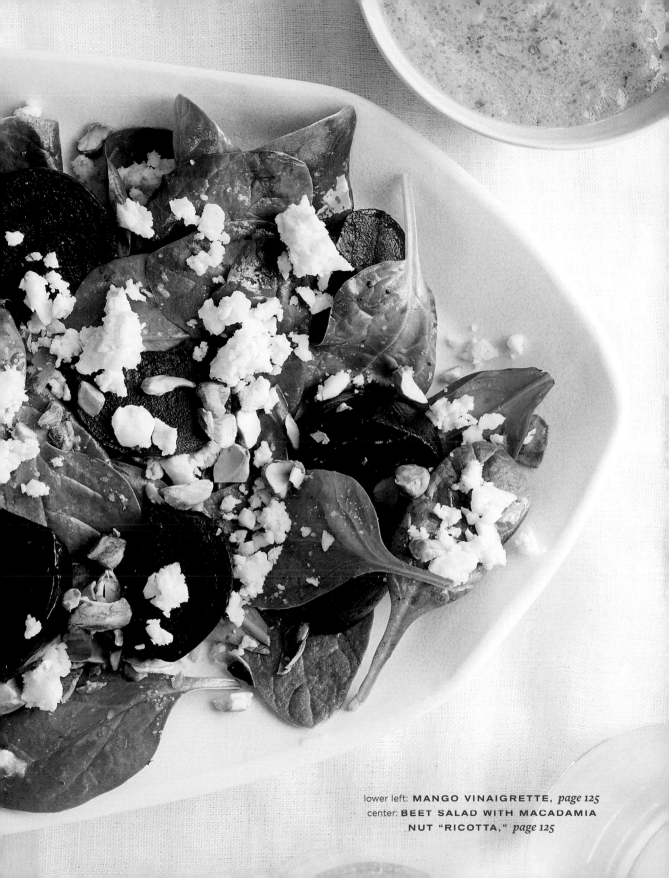

lower left: **MANGO VINAIGRETTE,** *page 125*
center: **BEET SALAD WITH MACADAMIA NUT "RICOTTA,"** *page 125*

GREEK SALAD
with Chickpeas

**SERVES 2 AS AN ENTRÉE
OR 4 AS A SIDE**
Prep and Cook Time
(with dried chickpeas):
1 hour, plus an overnight
soak for the chickpeas

Prep Time
(with canned chickpeas):
10 minutes

¼ cup dried chickpeas, or ½ cup
canned chickpeas, rinsed and
drained (see Note)
Finely ground Celtic salt
7 ounces romaine lettuce hearts,
chopped coarsely
¾ cup chopped English cucumber
10 to 12 pitted kalamata olives, rinsed
10 to 12 grape tomatoes, halved
1 tablespoon olive oil
¼ cup crumbled feta cheese

Most Greek salads are made with vinegar, which is too acidic and therefore too inflammatory, and raw onion is typically a main ingredient as well. Our solution is a straightforward olive oil–based dressing with a touch of Celtic salt.

1   To cook the dried chickpeas, place them in a large glass bowl, cover with water, and soak overnight. The next morning, drain and rinse them thoroughly. In a medium saucepan over high heat, combine the soaked and drained chickpeas with 2 cups of salted water, bring the water to a boil over high heat, then reduce the heat to medium. Cover and simmer for 40 to 45 minutes, until the chickpeas are tender but before they start falling apart. Drain and cool to room temperature.

2   Combine the chickpeas, lettuce, cucumber, olives, tomatoes, olive oil, and feta in a salad bowl and toss to coat all the ingredients with olive oil. Season with a pinch of salt. Divide the salad between two plates for an entrée or four plates for a side dish, and serve.

NOTE   If you're using canned chickpeas, skip to step 2.

BEET SALAD
with Macadamia Nut "Ricotta" and Mango Vinaigrette

SERVES 2

Prep and Cook Time: 2 hours, plus an overnight soak for the macadamia nuts

---

BEETS
2 medium beets, washed
4 fresh thyme sprigs

MACADAMIA NUT "RICOTTA"
½ cup raw unsalted macadamia nuts, soaked overnight
¼ cup almond milk or other nondairy milk
½ teaspoon finely ground Celtic salt

MANGO VINAIGRETTE
1 cup peeled and chopped ripe mango (about 1 mango)
2 tablespoons filtered water
1 teaspoon olive oil
¼ teaspoon finely ground Celtic salt
2 tablespoons chopped fresh cilantro

SALAD
2 cups baby spinach
2 tablespoons chopped pistachios

Our fun with tree nuts continues with a plant-based salad, eschewing cheese for macadamia, to bring a distinct flavor and texture to this dish.

1 **COOK THE BEETS:** Preheat the oven to 400°F. Lay a double layer of aluminum foil on a baking sheet. Place the beets and thyme on top, then wrap them into a tightly sealed bundle. Bake for 1 to 1½ hours, or until a fork slides easily through the beets. Remove from the oven. Unwrap the beets and let them cool slightly, then gently rub the beets with paper towels to remove their skins. Slice the beets into quarters and set them aside.

2 **MAKE THE "RICOTTA":** Meanwhile, rinse and drain the macadamia nuts, then place them in the bowl of a food processor. Add the almond milk and salt. Process until the mixture is creamy but still retains some texture, 1½ to 2 minutes. Transfer to a bowl, cover, and refrigerate until needed. Leftovers may be stored in the refrigerator for up to 3 days.

3 **MAKE THE VINAIGRETTE:** In the clean bowl of a food processor, combine the mango, filtered water, olive oil, and salt. Process until smooth, approximately 1 minute. Add the cilantro and pulse once or twice, until it speckles the dressing.

4 **ASSEMBLE THE SALAD:** Divide the spinach between two plates and top each with half the beets, the mango dressing, and the macadamia "ricotta." Garnish with chopped pistachios.

SPLIT PEA SOUP

SERVES 6 TO 8

Prep and Cook Time: 1½ hours,
plus more for cooling

---

2 tablespoons olive oil

1 medium leek, white parts only,
cleaned and sliced into rings

1 parsnip, peeled and coarsely
chopped

2 ounces turnip, peeled and cubed

4 ounces rutabaga, peeled and cubed

4 ounces celery root, peeled and
cubed

1 medium carrot, peeled and
shredded

1 (1-inch) piece fresh ginger, peeled
and grated

2 teaspoons coarsely ground
Celtic salt

¼ teaspoon ground cloves

1 teaspoon asafetida (see Kitchen
Note)

1 tablespoon fresh parsley leaves,
chopped

1 cup split peas

2 fresh bay leaves, or 1 dried

KITCHEN NOTE Asafetida is a spice
extracted from a fennel-like plant in the
mountains of Afghanistan and an ubiquitous
flavor enhancer in vegetarian dishes. The
spice has an uninviting odor, which recedes
completely in the heat of cooking, and
acquires a subtle flavor reminiscent of
sautéed onion and garlic.

Split pea soup is a universal staple of winter comfort
foods, and this Acid Watcher–friendly recipe offers all
the depth of flavor and texture without animal-based
products or acid-generating aromatics. You'll need either
an immersion or countertop blender to puree the soup.
If you are using a countertop version, make sure that the
soup has cooled to room temperature and, for best results,
puree it in batches. The soup tastes best when it is still
a touch chunky. It thickens in the refrigerator, so add as
much water as you need when reheating.

1   In a heavy-bottomed pot, preferably a Dutch oven,
heat the olive oil over medium-high heat. One at a
time and at 3- to 5-minute intervals, add and sauté
the leek, parsnip, turnip, rutabaga, celery root, and
carrot. Add splashes of water to prevent the veggies
from sticking, and stir frequently to prevent burning.

2   Add the ginger, salt, cloves, asafetida, and parsley
leaves and sauté for another 5 minutes. Don't worry
about overcooking the vegetables; just make sure
you keep them moist by adding water as needed.

3   Add the split peas, bay leaves, and 6 cups of water,
and bring to a boil on high heat. Reduce the heat to
low and skim the surface. Simmer the soup, partially
covered, for 45 minutes, stirring occasionally to
prevent clumping.

4   Allow the soup to come to room temperature.
Remove the bay leaves. Using an immersion or
countertop blender, puree the soup until it reaches
your desired consistency. Adjust the seasoning.
Reheat the soup fully to serve piping hot.

QUINOA TABBOULEH

SERVES 2
Prep and Cook Time: 35 minutes

½ cup white quinoa, rinsed
½ teaspoon finely ground Celtic salt
2 teaspoons lemon zest
1 cup chopped English cucumber
½ cup quartered grape tomatoes
¼ cup chopped fresh parsley
1 teaspoon olive oil
1 teaspoon ground sumac

This protein- and fiber-rich Mediterranean classic is traditionally made with lemon juice and raw scallions, which are both bothersome to the Acid Watcher. Here we've made fresh parsley the star and replaced acidic lemon juice with its more alkaline counterpart, lemon zest. If you're on the Maintenance Phase of the diet, you will greatly enjoy the addition of fresh tomato!

1   In a small saucepan, combine the quinoa and ¾ cup of water. Over high heat, bring the water to a boil. Immediately cover with a tight-fitting lid, and reduce the heat to the lowest setting. Cook for about 12 minutes, or until all of the liquid has been absorbed. Leaving the lid on, remove the saucepan from the heat and let it rest for 3 minutes.

2   Transfer the cooked quinoa to a large bowl, and add ¼ teaspoon of the salt and the lemon zest. Stir to allow the steam to escape, then let cool for 5 minutes.

3   To the cooled quinoa, add the cucumber, tomato, parsley, olive oil, sumac, and the remaining ¼ teaspoon salt. Stir to combine. Serve immediately. Leftovers may be covered and stored in the refrigerator for up to 2 days.

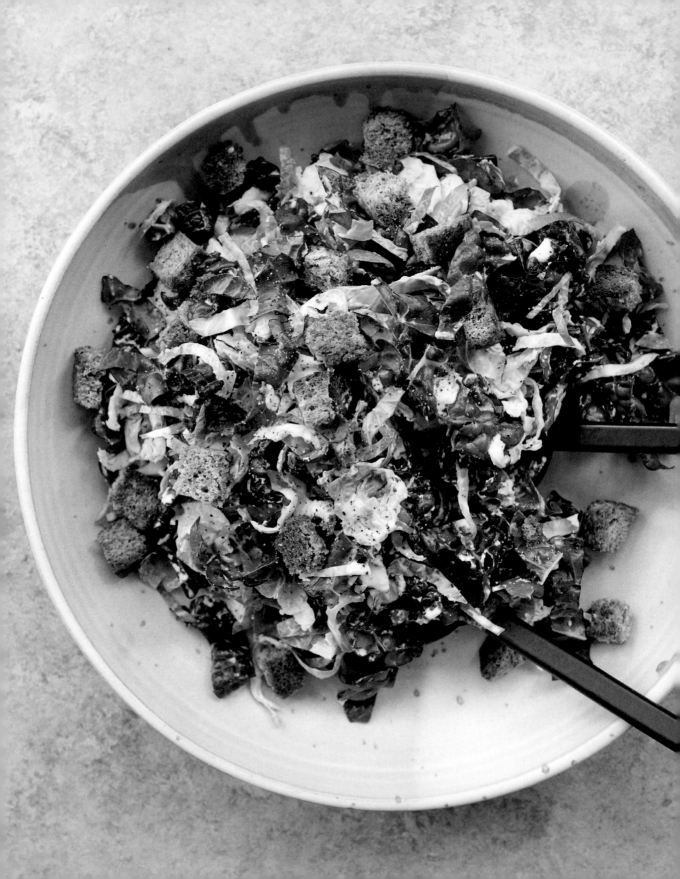

Kale and Brussels
CAESAR SALAD

SERVES 2

Prep and Cook Time: 30 minutes,
plus an overnight soak for the cashews

CROUTONS

2 slices Ezekiel 4:9 Sprouted Whole
Grain Bread, cubed

1½ teaspoons olive oil

⅛ teaspoon finely ground Celtic salt

CAESAR DRESSING

½ cup raw unsalted cashews, soaked
overnight

6 tablespoons filtered water

2 teaspoons apple cider vinegar

¾ teaspoon finely ground
Celtic salt

1 tablespoon lemon zest
(zest of 1 lemon)

SALAD

2 cups thinly sliced curly, lacinato, or
purple kale

½ teaspoon olive oil

¼ teaspoon finely ground Celtic salt

2 cups thinly sliced Brussels sprouts

The Acid Watcher version of Caesar dressing is plant-based, using cashews in both the egg and Parmesan roles. Cashews also neutralize the apple cider vinegar enough to make this applicable during the Healing Phase. This dressing has widespread uses beyond just on greens; use as a creamy dressing to enhance fish or on a variety of sandwiches.

1   MAKE THE CROUTONS: Preheat the oven to 375°F. On a small baking sheet, toss the bread cubes with the olive oil and salt. Bake for about 10 minutes, or until crisp and lightly browned. Set aside.

2   MAKE THE DRESSING: In the meantime, rinse and drain the cashews. Place them in a blender, along with the filtered water, vinegar, salt, and lemon zest. Blend on high for 2 to 3 minutes, until completely creamy. Refrigerate until needed. Leftover dressing may be stored in the refrigerator for up to 4 days.

3   PREPARE THE SALAD: In a large bowl, combine the sliced kale, olive oil, and salt. Massage the kale until it turns a deep green color and begins to wilt, about 30 seconds. Add the sliced Brussels sprouts. Add the croutons and 3 tablespoons of the dressing. Toss to combine and serve immediately. Add more dressing, if desired.

SPINACH AND GRILLED ASIAN PEAR SALAD

with Sesame Dressing

SERVES 2

Prep and Cook Time: 15 minutes

1 tablespoon olive oil
1 Asian pear, cored and sliced
¼ inch thick

SESAME DRESSING
2 tablespoons tahini
2 tablespoons filtered water
1 tablespoon tamari
1 teaspoon manuka honey
1 teaspoon distilled white vinegar

SALAD
4 cups baby spinach
½ cup chopped English cucumber
½ cup shredded carrot
(approximately 1 carrot)
1 tablespoon white or black
sesame seeds

The counterpoint to this salad is a tangy sesame dressing in which the tahini neutralizes the distilled white vinegar.

1   Warm a grill pan over high heat and brush it with olive oil. Grill the sliced pear until you see grill marks, about 1 minute on each side. Set aside.

2   **MAKE THE DRESSING:** Combine the tahini, filtered water, tamari, honey, and vinegar in a small bowl and whisk until smooth.

3   **ASSEMBLE THE SALAD:** Divide the spinach evenly between two plates, creating a bed for the rest of the ingredients. Top with grilled Asian pear, chopped cucumber, and shredded carrot. Drizzle with sesame dressing, sprinkle with the sesame seeds, and serve.

APPLE, FENNEL, AND ARUGULA SALAD

SERVES 2 FOR A MAIN DISH OR 4 AS A SIDE

Prep and Cook Time: 20 minutes

½ cup chopped walnuts

2 medium apples, Gala, Golden Delicious, or a combination

1½ cups arugula

⅓ cup stringless pea shoots, cut crosswise into bite-size pieces

1 fennel bulb, cored, outer layer removed, and thinly sliced, fronds reserved

½ cup shredded Parmesan cheese

½ teaspoon coarsely ground Celtic salt

⅔ cup Weeknight Ambrosia Dressing (page 168)

Those who prefer seasonal produce for their salads complain about the paucity of available fresh vegetables in the fall, which tends to be limited to starchy root vegetables, winter squash, and sturdy lettuces. However, we see plenty of delicious opportunities for fresh salads when the weather turns, especially when fall vegetables are combined with fruit and nuts.

1   In a small heavy-bottomed skillet set over high heat, toast the walnuts for 3 to 5 minutes, turning the walnuts with a wooden or silicone spoon as needed to prevent them from burning. Don't walk away; walnuts can burn quickly. Place two-thirds of the walnuts into a large mixing bowl and let cool for 2 to 3 minutes. Reserve the remaining walnuts in a separate bowl. (Don't leave them in the skillet, as they will continue toasting from the heat of the pan.)

2   While the walnuts are cooling, core and slice the apples into matchsticks. Place them in the bowl with the walnuts. Add the arugula, pea shoots, sliced fennel, half the fennel fronds, half the Parmesan cheese, and the salt. Mix to combine.

3   Add the dressing, in batches, and continue to mix the salad thoroughly. Place the salad into serving bowls and top with the remaining Parmesan cheese, the toasted walnuts, and the remaining fennel fronds. Serve immediately.

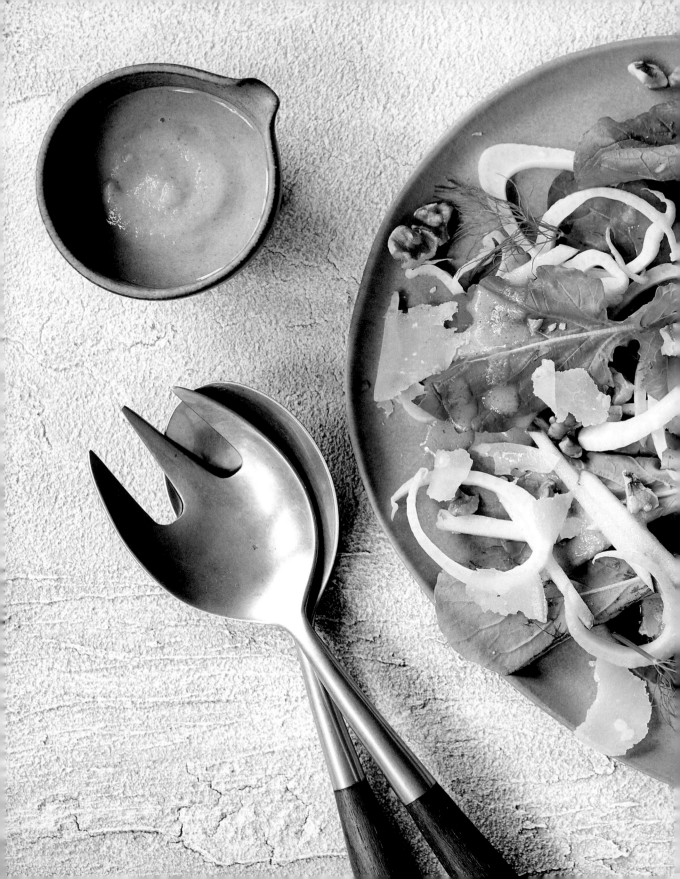

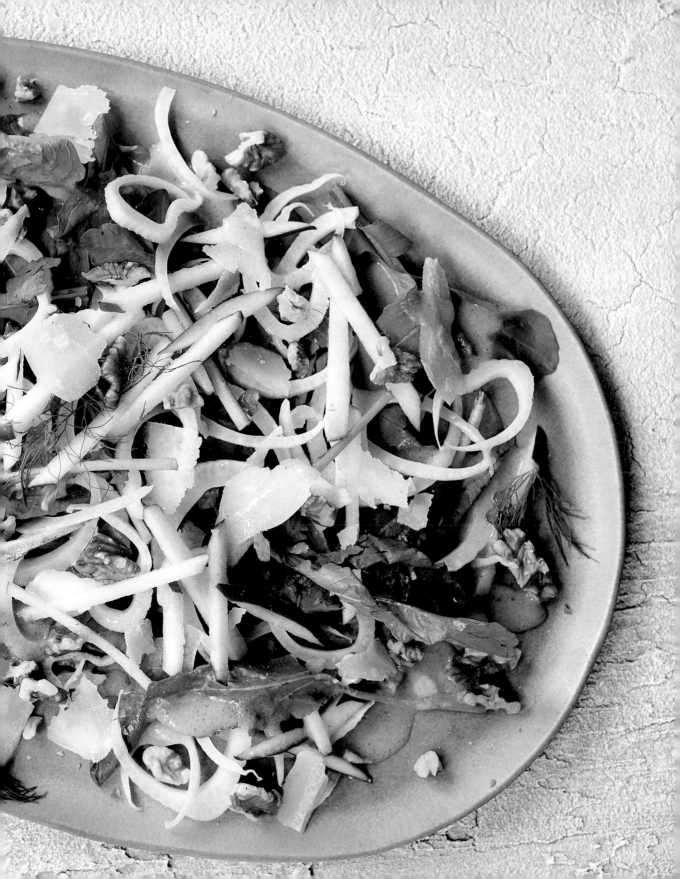

THE MAIN
EVENTS

H HEALING PHASE   M MAINTENANCE PHASE

Pan-Seared
FALAFEL

SERVES 2; MAKES 8 FALAFEL

Prep and Cook Time: 30 minutes, plus an overnight soak for the chickpeas

½ cup dried chickpeas, soaked overnight (see Kitchen Note)

¼ cup chopped fresh parsley

¼ cup chopped fresh cilantro

½ teaspoon ground cumin

1 teaspoon ground sumac

½ teaspoon finely ground Celtic salt

2 teaspoons olive oil

Real Hummus (page 87), Magra's Baba (Baba Ghanouj) (page 88), and/or Tzatziki Sauce (page 173), for serving (optional)

Traditionally, "falafel stand" falafel is a deep-fried treat. By pan-searing the falafel instead, this plant-based savory dish becomes a healthy dinner. It can be accompanied by hummus, baba ghanouj, or tzatziki.

1   Rinse and drain the soaked chickpeas.

2   In the bowl of a food processor, combine the chickpeas, parsley, cilantro, cumin, sumac, and salt. Process until the mixture is finely minced, about 1 minute. It shouldn't be totally smooth; it needs to hold together when squeezed. If it does crumble, pulse the mixture a few more times. Transfer the mixture to a bowl and refrigerate for 10 minutes to set.

3   Form the chickpea mixture into eight 1- to 2-inch patties.

4   In a large pan over medium-high heat, warm the olive oil. Sear the falafel in 2 batches of 4 for about 4 minutes, until golden brown. Flip and sear for another 2 minutes. Serve the falafel warm with your choice of sauces, if desired.

KITCHEN NOTE   Do not use canned chickpeas as they are fully cooked and will result in a mushy falafel.

GRILLED SALMON
with Crispy Skin

SERVES 2

Prep and Cook Time: 15 minutes

2 (6-ounce) wild salmon fillets,
  skin on
Coarsely ground Celtic salt
1 tablespoon olive oil

A good piece of wild salmon does not require much adornment to bring out its full flavor. One way to "spice" up salmon is to crisp the skin, which is full of healthy omega-3 fats.

1   Pat the salmon fillets dry on both sides with a paper towel and season both sides with Celtic salt.

2   In a nonstick grill pan set over high heat, heat the olive oil until very hot, about 4 minutes. Place the salmon in the pan, skin side down, and reduce the heat to medium-high. With the back of a spatula, press firmly on the fish for the first minute of cooking. Cook for another 4 minutes, making 5 minutes total, skin side down (this timing works very well for a 1-inch-thick fillet, but you may need to cook these longer if they're thicker). The fish should be about 90 percent cooked; flip it with the spatula and turn the heat off, letting the heat of the pan cook the fish for 1 more minute, or until the internal temperature reaches 120°F on an instant-read thermometer.

3   Place the fillets on a paper towel to drain any excess oil, then transfer them to plates and serve.

VEGGIE BURGER

MAKES 4 PATTIES
Prep and Cook Time: 1½ hours

1 medium red beet (about 4 ounces)
1½ teaspoons olive oil
4 button mushrooms, chopped
1¼ teaspoons finely ground Celtic salt
¾ cup cooked brown rice
2 tablespoons chopped walnuts
1 tablespoon flaxseed meal
1 large egg, whisked
2 tablespoons chopped fresh parsley
8 slices lightly toasted Ezekiel
  Sprouted Whole Grain bread,
  for serving
4 tablespoons Caesar Dressing
  (page 129), for serving
¼ English cucumber, sliced (12 slices),
  for serving
Sliced avocado, for serving

This flavorful, savory beet-based patty has nary a processed ingredient. To complete the meal combine this burger with Ezekiel bread, avocado, cucumber, and our Acid Watcher Caesar dressing.

1   Preheat the oven to 400°F. Lay a double layer of aluminum foil on a baking sheet. Place the beet on top, then wrap it into a tightly sealed bundle. Bake for about 1 hour, or until a fork slides through the beet easily. Unwrap and let cool slightly, then gently rub it with paper towels to remove the skin. Chop the beet and set it aside; you should have about ¾ cup.

2   In the meantime, heat ½ teaspoon of the olive oil in a small pan over medium heat. Add the mushrooms and ¼ teaspoon of the salt, and sauté until lightly golden, about 5 minutes.

3   In the bowl of a food processor, combine the brown rice, chopped beet, mushrooms, walnuts, flaxseed meal, egg, parsley, and the remaining 1 teaspoon salt. Pulse to a coarsely ground texture, about 30 seconds, then remove three-fourths of the mixture. Process the rest of the mixture until smooth, and stir it into the coarse mixture until thoroughly mixed. Refrigerate for 10 minutes to set.

4   Divide the mixture into 4 equal portions and form each into a patty about ½ inch thick. In a medium pan over medium-low heat, warm the remaining 1 teaspoon of olive oil and sear the patties for about 5 minutes per side, until golden brown and crispy.

5   Serve the patties on lightly toasted Ezekiel bread with Caesar dressing, sliced cucumber, and avocado.

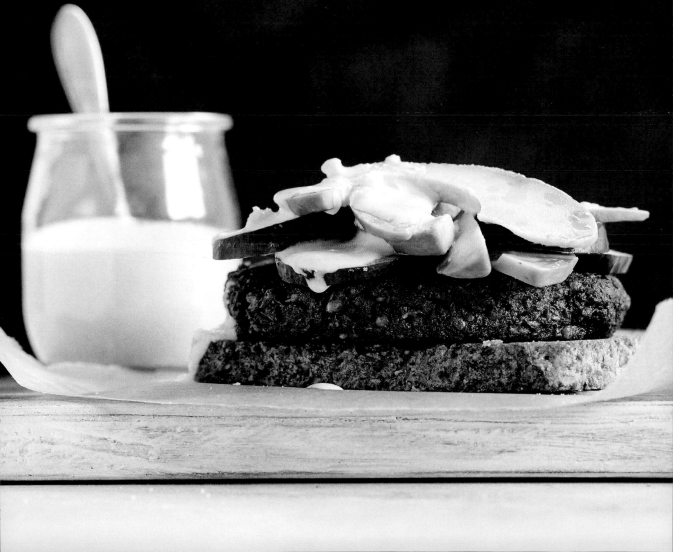

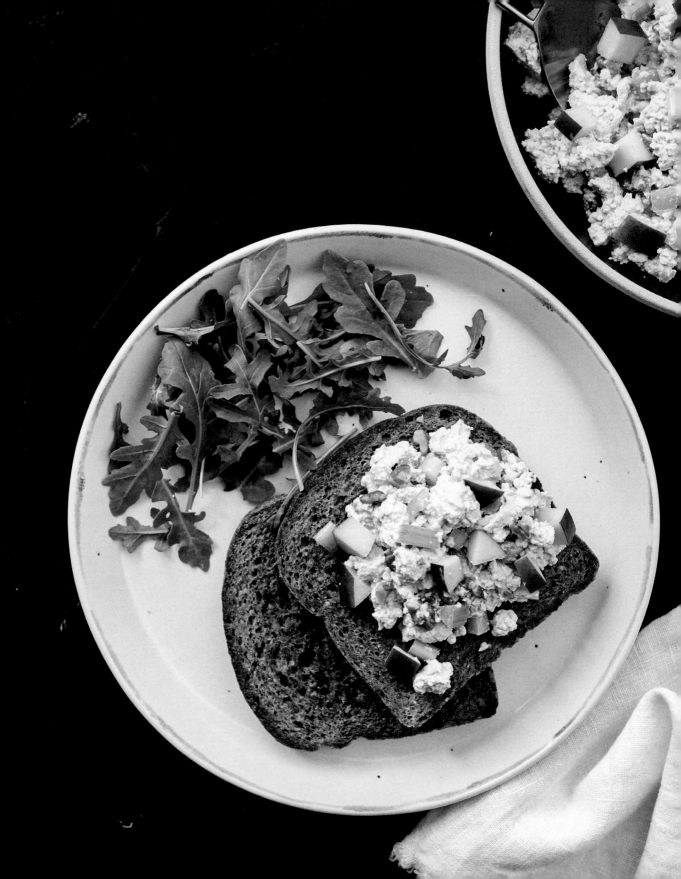

TOFU WALDORF SALAD

SERVES 2
Prep time: 15 minutes

---

1 (14-ounce) block firm tofu

1 tablespoon eggless mayonnaise, preferably Primal Kitchen

¼ teaspoon sweet paprika

Pinch of ground turmeric

¼ teaspoon coarsely ground Celtic salt

½ cup diced celery, approximately 1 stalk

½ cup diced Gala apple

¼ cup coarsely chopped walnuts

1 to 2 cups arugula—1 cup if having the tofu mixture on toasted whole-grain bread; 2 cups if having the tofu mixture just on a bed of arugula

2 slices whole-grain bread (optional), preferably Bread Alone Nine Mixed Grain bread

Our Tofu Waldorf is plant-based, where the "mayo" we use is an eggless, plant-based spread whose relative acidity is neutralized by the tofu. The added spices can act as carminatives, and the Gala apple is between pH 4 and 5, so this is a Maintenance Phase dish.

1   Drain and rinse the tofu and then pat it well with paper towels to remove any excess moisture. Cut the tofu into 8 large chunks and place them in a medium bowl. Using the back of a fork, mash the chunks of tofu so that the mixture takes on the traditional crumbly texture of egg salad.

2   Add mayo, spices, and salt to the tofu and mix and mash the mixture with your fork to incorporate everything. Add the celery, apple, and walnuts to the bowl, and stir to combine.

3   Serve on a bed of arugula or, if desired, open-faced on toasted whole-grain bread, topped with the arugula.

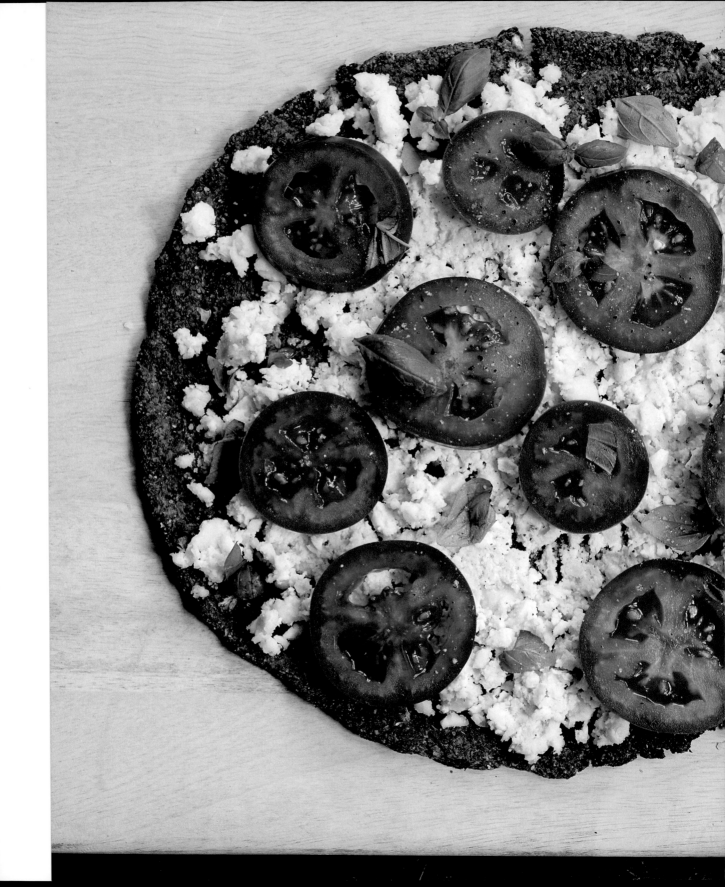

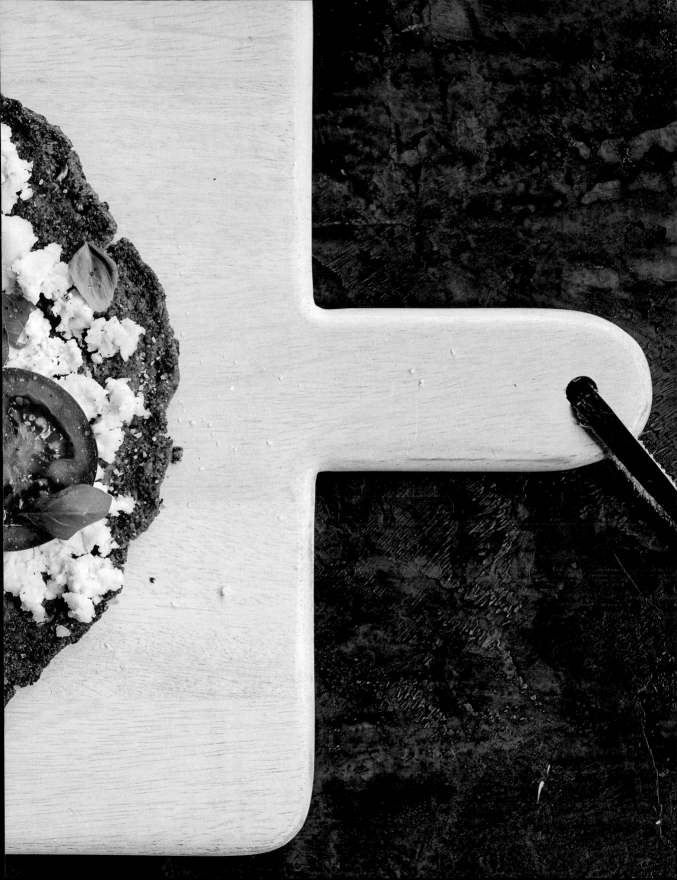

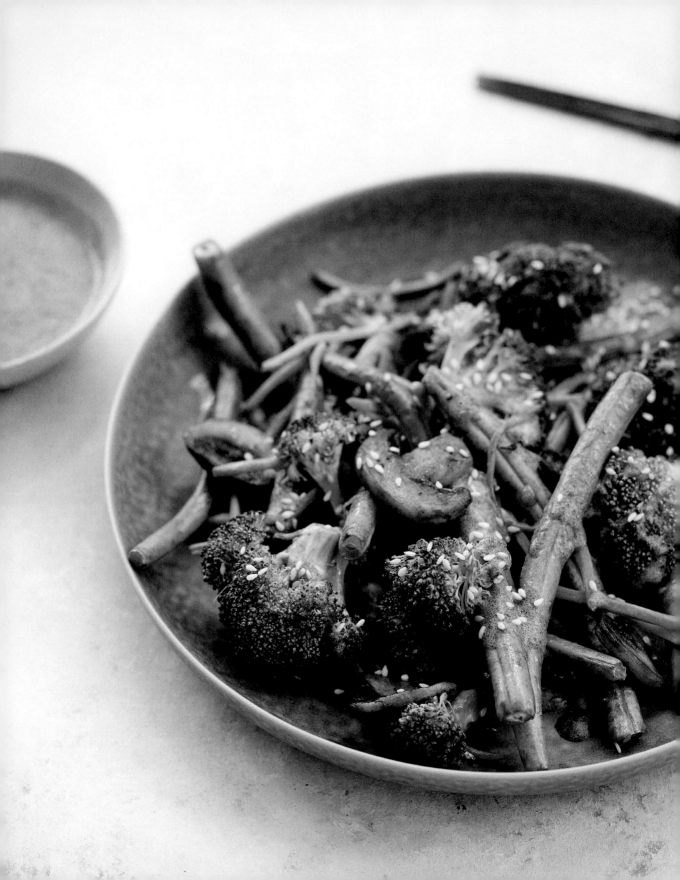

VEGGIE STIR-FRY
in Brown Sauce

SERVES 2

Prep and Cook Time: 25 minutes

BROWN SAUCE

¼ cup tamari
6 tablespoons filtered water
8 pitted Deglet dates (about
  2½ ounces pitted)

VEGGIES
2 teaspoons olive oil
1 cup whole green beans, ends
  trimmed
1 cup broccoli florets
1 cup sliced button mushrooms
½ cup sliced or shredded carrots
1 teaspoon toasted sesame seeds

Generally, tamari is a gluten-free but more alkaline (above pH 5) version of soy sauce, and it doesn't have the added sugar of teriyaki sauce.

1   **MAKE THE BROWN SAUCE:** In a blender, combine the tamari, filtered water, and dates. Blend until thickened and smooth, 1 to 2 minutes. (This recipe makes about ½ cup; whatever is left over can be stored in an airtight container in the refrigerator for up to 5 days.)

2   **STIR-FRY THE VEGGIES:** Heat the olive oil in a large frying pan over medium-high heat. Add the green beans, broccoli, mushrooms, and carrots, and stir. Cover and cook for 5 to 6 minutes, until the vegetables are tender but still slightly crunchy.

3   Remove the pan from the heat and toss in ¼ cup of the sauce; stir. Sprinkle with the sesame seeds and serve. Top with more sauce, if desired.

Butternut Squash "MAC 'N' CHEESE"

SERVES 2
Prep and Cook Time: 40 minutes

¾ cup peeled and cubed butternut squash

⅛ cup raw unsalted cashews

¼ cup chopped sweet onion

8 ounces gluten-free elbow "macaroni," preferably Ancient Harvest Pasta Elbows containing corn and quinoa

½ teaspoon coarsely ground Celtic salt

Pinch of sweet paprika

Pinch of ground turmeric

Pinch of ground nutmeg

½ tablespoon fresh lemon juice

½ teaspoon Dijon mustard

Comfort food that won't make you feel uncomfortable? By eliminating dairy and gluten and substituting cashews and organic quinoa and corn, respectively, and cooking the onion, traditional macaroni and cheese now has an Acid Watcher Maintenance Phase version.

1   Place the butternut squash, cashews, and onions in a medium saucepan and add enough water to cover by 1 inch. Bring the water to a boil over high heat and then reduce the heat to low. Cook for about 15 minutes, or until the vegetables are tender.

2   While the vegetables and nuts are cooking, prepare the pasta according to the package instructions. Drain any water and set the pasta aside, covered to keep warm.

3   When the vegetables are done, drain, saving ⅛ cup of the cooking water.

4   To make the sauce, combine the butternut squash mixture, reserved cooking water, salt, spices, lemon juice, and mustard in a blender and blend on high until completely creamy, about 1 minute.

5   Add the sauce to the pot with the cooked pasta, stir to combine, and reheat over low heat. Serve immediately.

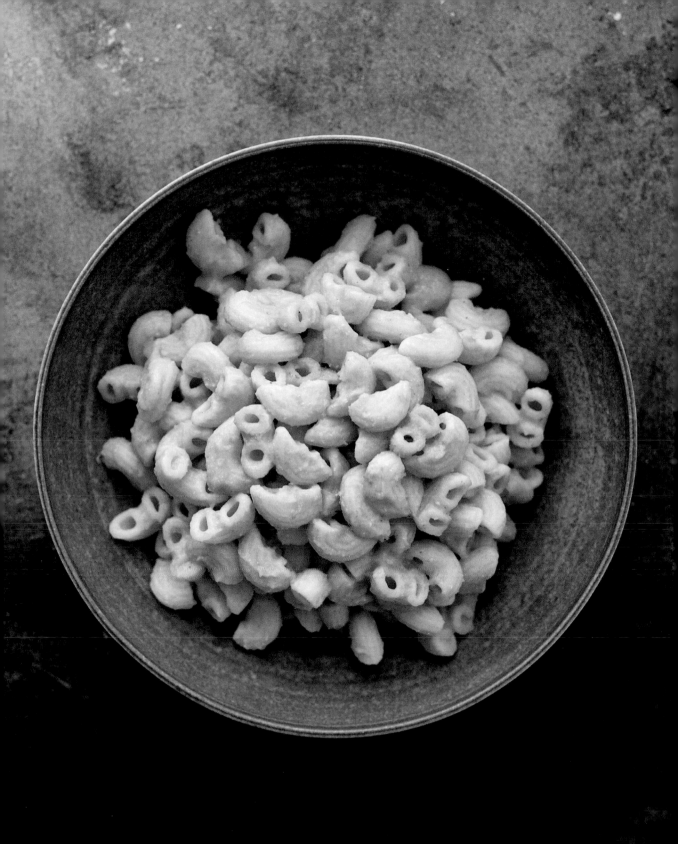

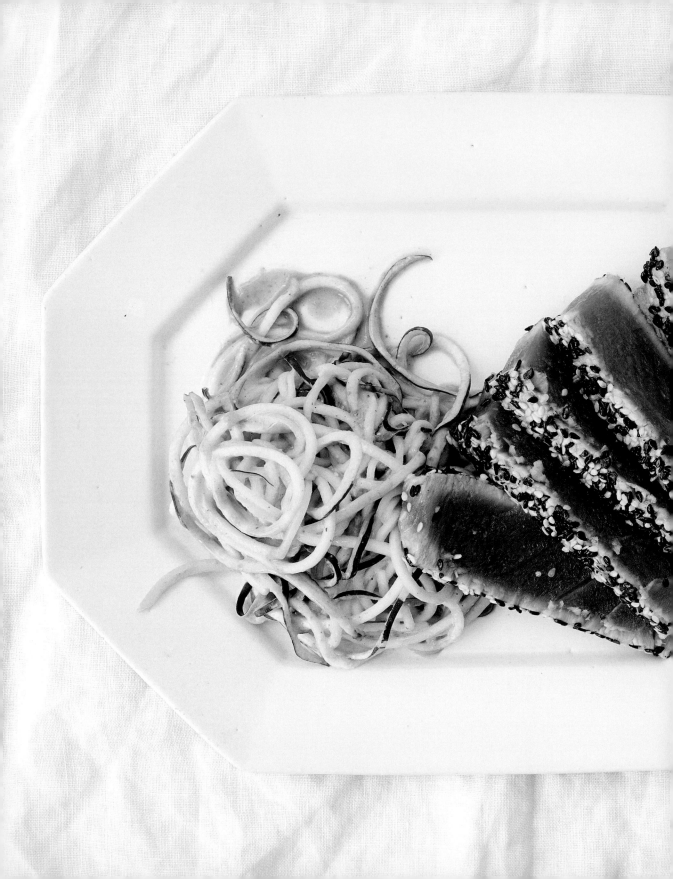

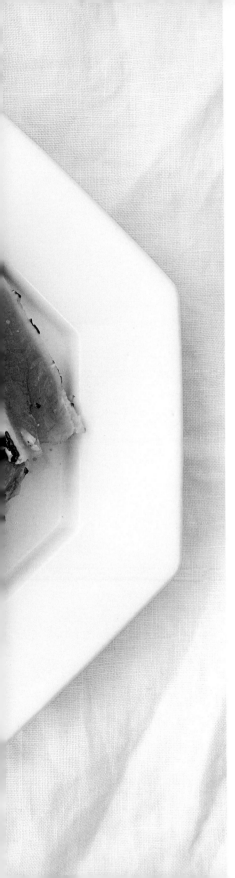

SESAME-CRUSTED TUNA
with Zoodles and Peanut Sauce

SERVES 2
Prep and Cook Time: 30 minutes

The sauce for the zoodles is the Acid Watcher–friendly version of traditional peanut sauce, a staple of many a Chinese take-out food fest. You can always serve the zoodles with the peanut sauce, without the tuna, as a side dish. As an accompaniment to the tuna, any of our veggie side dishes would also pair well.

Peanut Sauce (page 176)
6 cups spiralized zucchini zoodles
2 tablespoons white sesame seeds
2 tablespoons black sesame seeds
2 (6-ounce) wild tuna steaks
1 teaspoon olive oil
Coarsely ground Celtic salt

1   In a large bowl, toss the peanut sauce with the zoodles. Set aside.

2   In a shallow baking dish, mix together the sesame seeds. Coat both sides of each tuna steak with the seeds.

3   In a large skillet over medium-high heat, heat the olive oil. When it is hot, sear the tuna for 2 minutes on each side, or to the desired level of doneness.

4   Remove the tuna from the pan, sprinkle it evenly with salt, slice it, and serve over the zoodles.

Mediterranean
MONKFISH WITH OLIVES

SERVES 2

Prep and Cook Time: 35 minutes

---

2 teaspoons olive oil

2 (6-ounce) monkfish fillets

10 pitted black kalamata olives, plus some of the brine

1 teaspoon lemon zest

2 tablespoons chopped beefsteak tomato or tomatoes on the vine

1 teaspoon capers in salt

Coarsely ground Celtic salt

Monkfish is full of micronutrients and relatively low in mercury. There shouldn't be any concern about the acidity of vinegar in the olive brine, as it will burn away during the cooking process.

1   Preheat the oven to 475°F.

2   Coat the bottom of a small baking dish with the olive oil and place the fish fillets in the dish. Top each fish fillet with the olives, lemon zest, chopped tomatoes, capers, and a generous spoonful of olive brine. Sprinkle each with a pinch of Celtic salt.

3   Bake for about 27 minutes, or until the fish flakes easily with a fork. Serve immediately.

COCONUT SHRIMP

SERVES 2

Prep and Cook Time: 25 minutes

½ cup almond flour

½ cup unsweetened shredded coconut

½ teaspoon finely ground Celtic salt

20 medium shrimp, cleaned

1 large egg, whisked

2 tablespoons coconut oil

Mango Vinaigrette (page 125), for serving (optional)

Peanut Sauce (page 176), for serving (optional)

Our coconut shrimp is a quick, easy-to-prepare, and delicious recipe that substitutes almond flour for regular wheat flour and sautés instead of deep-fries the shrimp. Any number of dipping sauces (our favorites are mentioned below) go beautifully with this dish.

1   In a large shallow bowl, combine the almond flour, shredded coconut, and salt. Dip each of the shrimp in the whisked egg and then into the almond-flour mixture. Make sure the shrimp are very well coated in the flour mixture. Set aside.

2   In a large skillet set over medium-high heat, melt 1 tablespoon of the coconut oil. Add half of the coated shrimp to the skillet and sauté for 2 minutes without stirring. (Do not attempt to sauté all 20 shrimp in one batch or you will overcrowd the pan and the shrimp will steam, not sauté!) Using tongs, flip each shrimp by its tail and sauté the other side for 1 more minute, then reduce the heat to low and sauté for another minute. Place the sautéed shrimp on paper towels to drain while you cook the remaining shrimp.

3   Clean the pan well with water and a paper towel and repeat the same process with the remaining 10 shrimp and coconut oil. Transfer the coconut shrimp to plates and serve with your choice of dipping sauces; we like mango vinaigrette and peanut sauce.

Grilled

FISH TACOS

SERVES 2

Prep and Cook Time: 25 minutes

SLAW

3 cups shredded white cabbage or a mix of white and red cabbage

3 tablespoons Caesar Dressing (page 129), plus more (optional) for serving

MARINADE

1 tablespoon olive oil

1 tablespoon fresh lime juice

½ teaspoon ground cumin

½ teaspoon ground coriander

½ teaspoon sweet paprika

¼ teaspoon finely ground Celtic salt

2 (6-ounce) tilapia fillets

Olive oil, for the grill pan

4 corn tortillas, preferably Trader Joe's Corn Tortillas or Ezekiel 4:9 Sprouted Corn Tortillas

⅓ cup chopped mango

1 Hass avocado, peeled, pitted, and cubed

2 tablespoons coarsely chopped fresh cilantro

These fish tacos use tilapia, which is a tasty, mild (that is, non-fishy), protein-packed fish. Like most types of fish, wild-caught tilapia is much healthier to eat than the more common farmed tilapia. However, if farmed under strict rules and guidelines, such as those followed by the Regal Springs company (regalsprings.com), it doesn't have many of the dangers of farmed fish. Regal Springs is certified by the Aquaculture Stewardship Council (ASC), which has been auditing and certifying farm-raised tilapia for several years to ensure safety standards for farmed tilapia.

1   **MAKE THE SLAW:** In a medium bowl, toss the shredded cabbage with the dressing. Cover and refrigerate until ready to serve.

2   **MAKE THE MARINADE:** In a large shallow bowl, whisk together the olive oil, lime juice, spices, and salt. Place the tilapia in the marinade and coat the fillets evenly on both sides. Let them marinate while you preheat the pan.

3   Brush a nonstick grill pan with 1 teaspoon of olive oil and heat it over medium-high heat. Remove the fish from the marinade and drain off any excess. Place the fish in the pan and cook for 3 minutes on each side, or until the fish flakes easily with a fork.

4   Divide small pieces of the fish evenly among the 4 corn tortillas and top each with one-fourth of the slaw, chopped mango, avocado, and cilantro. Drizzle with extra dressing, if desired, and serve immediately.

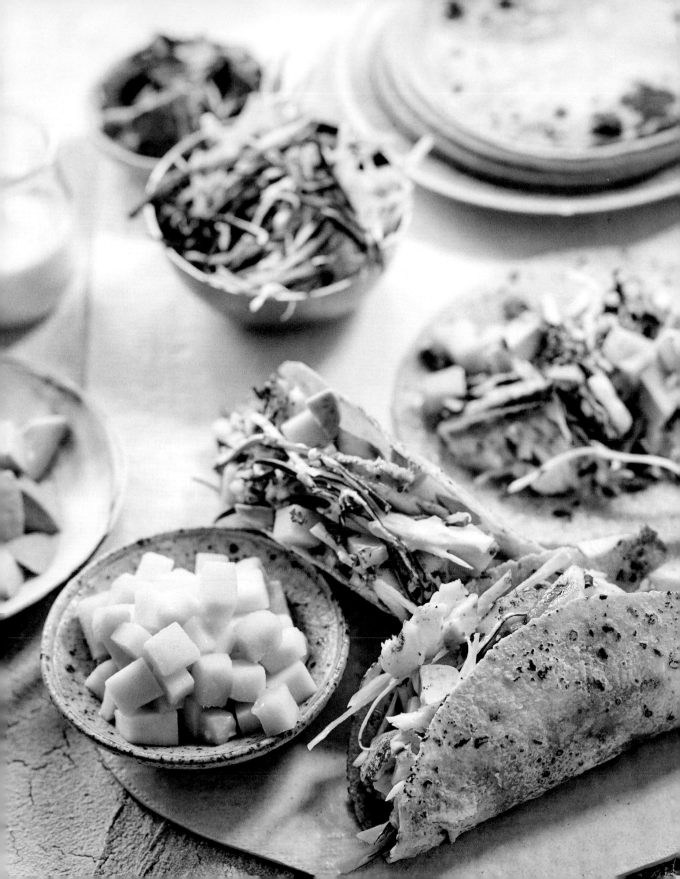

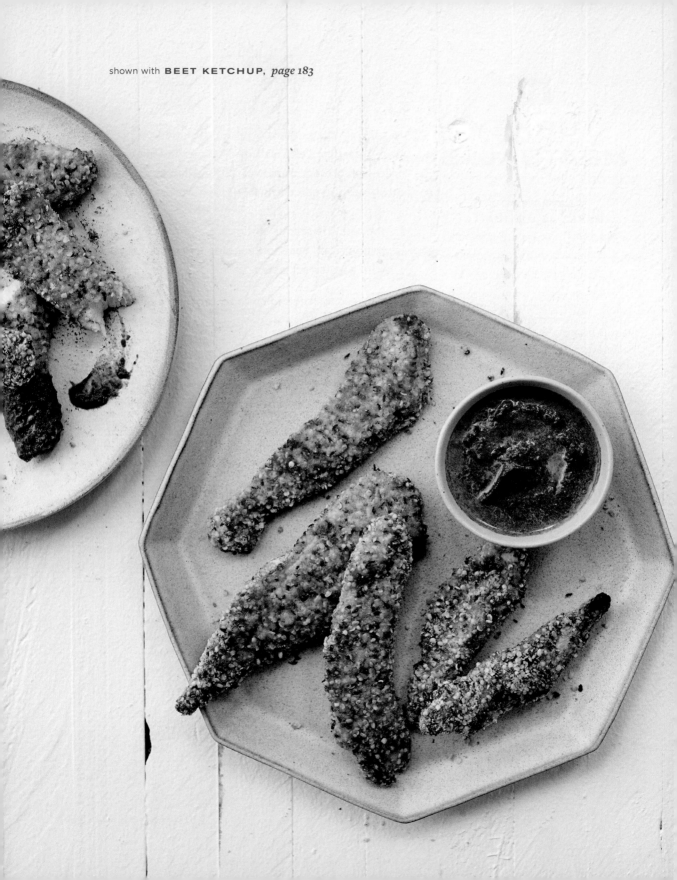
shown with **BEET KETCHUP,** *page 183*

GLUTEN-FREE "BREADED" CHICKEN TENDERS

with Hempseed and Almond Flour

SERVES 2
Prep and Cook Time: 35 minutes

¼ cup almond flour
¼ cup hempseeds
¼ teaspoon sweet paprika
¼ teaspoon ground cumin
½ teaspoon finely ground Celtic salt
1 large egg (optional; see Note)
2 (6-ounce) organic chicken breasts,
   cut into 6 or 7 pieces (tenders),
   lengthwise
Caesar Dressing (page 129) and/
   or Beet Ketchup (page 183), for
   serving (optional)

It is hard to believe that these tenders are all protein and entirely gluten- and oil-free. The hempseeds help to add a beautiful thick coating that in every way resembles a heart- and throat-burn-inducing deep-fried chicken tender.

1   Preheat the oven to 400°F. Line a large baking sheet with parchment paper.

2   In a shallow baking dish, create the "breading" by combining the almond flour, hempseeds, spices, and salt; mix thoroughly. In a small bowl, whisk the egg, if using; place it next to the breading dish.

3   Dip each chicken tender first into the egg, then transfer it to the baking dish with the "breading" mixture, coating each piece on all sides. Carefully place each "breaded" chicken tender on the parchment-lined sheet. Repeat until all the chicken is coated.

4   Bake the tenders for 20 to 25 minutes, until cooked through and the internal temperature reaches 165°F. Remove from the oven. Serve with Caesar dressing and/or beet ketchup, if desired.

NOTE For an egg-free version, just skip the egg and dip the chicken tenders directly into the breading mixture. It will still adhere to the chicken!

Ed's Sunday Night
WHOLE ROAST CHICKEN

SERVES 2 TO 4

Prep and Cook Time: 1¼ hours

1 (3½- to 4-pound) air-chilled organic chicken, fresh from the butcher

Coarsely ground Celtic salt

The perfect roast chicken should be tender, moist, crispy enough, easy to make, and predictable in every way. Most roast chicken calls for butter and basting, which isn't the healthiest option. This simple roast chicken requires no fussing once it's put into the oven, and the prep is simple and easy, too. It will quickly become your family's Sunday night fave. It's perfect salted with plain Celtic salt, but feel free to stuff the cavity with lemon slices and your favorite herbs if you wish. Serve with Steamed Asparagus with Shaved Parmesan (page 105) for a full meal!

1   Preheat the oven to 425°F (see Kitchen Note).

2   Rub all sides of the chicken with a generous amount of salt. Place the chicken, breast side up, in a roasting pan and cook for about 65 minutes, or until the internal temperature reaches 165°F. Remove from the oven. Let the chicken rest for 5 minutes before carving and serving.

KITCHEN NOTE Not all ovens will heat to the exact temperature you set them to. To make sure that you do not overcook the chicken; check with a meat thermometer after 1 hour. The chicken is done when the thermometer inserted into the deepest part of the thigh reads 165 degrees F.

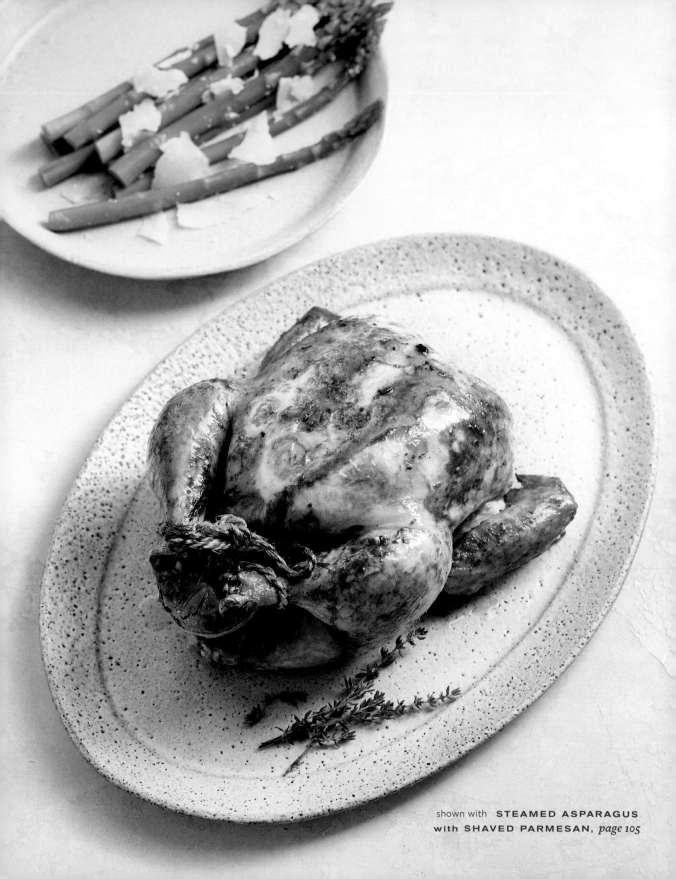

shown with **STEAMED ASPARAGUS**
with **SHAVED PARMESAN**, *page 105*

NEW OLD FAVORITES (DRESSINGS AND BASICS)

H HEALING PHASE   M MAINTENANCE PHASE

CREAMY DRESSING

YIELDS 1¼ CUPS

Prep Time: 10 minutes, plus an
overnight soak for cashews

1 cup raw unsalted cashews, soaked
 overnight (see Doctor's Note)
¾ cup filtered water
1 tablespoon olive oil
½ teaspoon Dijon mustard
5 teaspoons fresh lemon juice
½ teaspoon coarsely ground
 Celtic salt

This flavorful, slightly tangy dressing satisfies one's craving for a creamy dressing without any dairy. It is great not only on greens but also on sandwiches.

Drain and rinse cashews. Combine all the ingredients in a blender and blend on high speed for 2 to 3 minutes, until completely creamy.

DOCTOR'S NOTE This versatile Creamy Dressing epitomizes the acid neutralization ethos of this cookbook. Lemon juice and mustard are two of the most acidic substances one can consume, both at pH 3 or below. However, using cashews neutralizes the acidity essentially in two ways. Not only are cashews alkaline, but also, importantly, they are very concentrated or dense, so when applied in the volumes recommended, even very acidic foods can be pushed above pH 4 into Maintenance Phase territory.

BASIC
"Vinaigrette"

YIELDS ¼ CUP
Prep Time: 5 minutes

¼ cup olive oil
Zest of 2 lemons (see Doctor's Note)
½ teaspoon coarsely ground
   Celtic salt

In a small bowl, whisk together all the ingredients and place them in a sealable jar. Shake very well before serving. Refrigerate in an airtight container for up to 2 days.

DOCTOR'S NOTE My patients often say to me, "I'm so sad that I can't have salad anymore," because many feel a salad dressing must include vinegar and/or lemon. Vinegar (balsamic, apple cider, red wine, etc.) and lemon are both quite acidic, and Acid Watchers generally avoid them as primary ingredients in a dressing. To address the missing flavor that vinegar brings, we created a workhorse salad dressing that incorporates lemon zest and has widespread use in almost any salad, even in the Healing Phase.

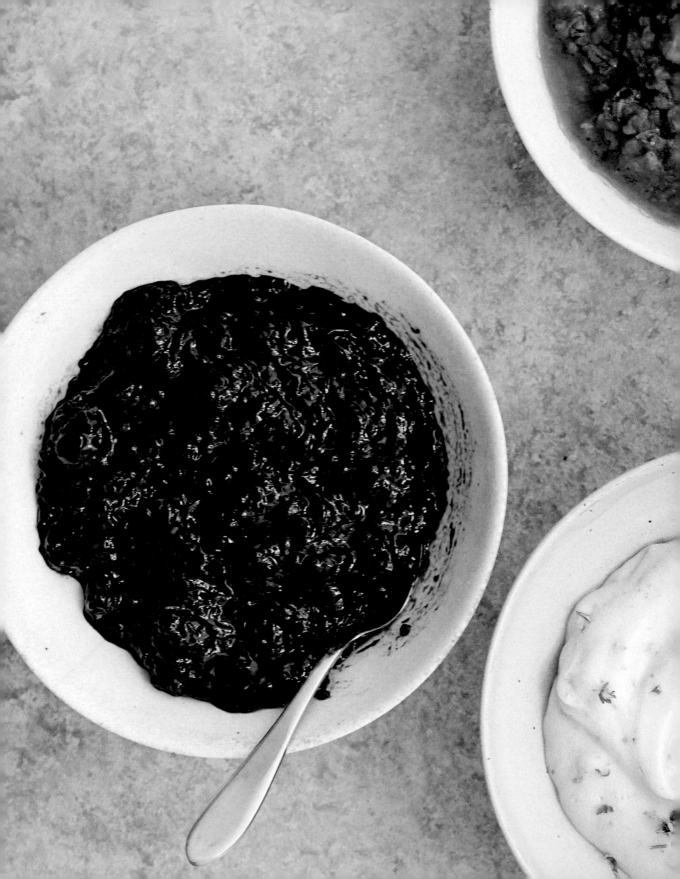

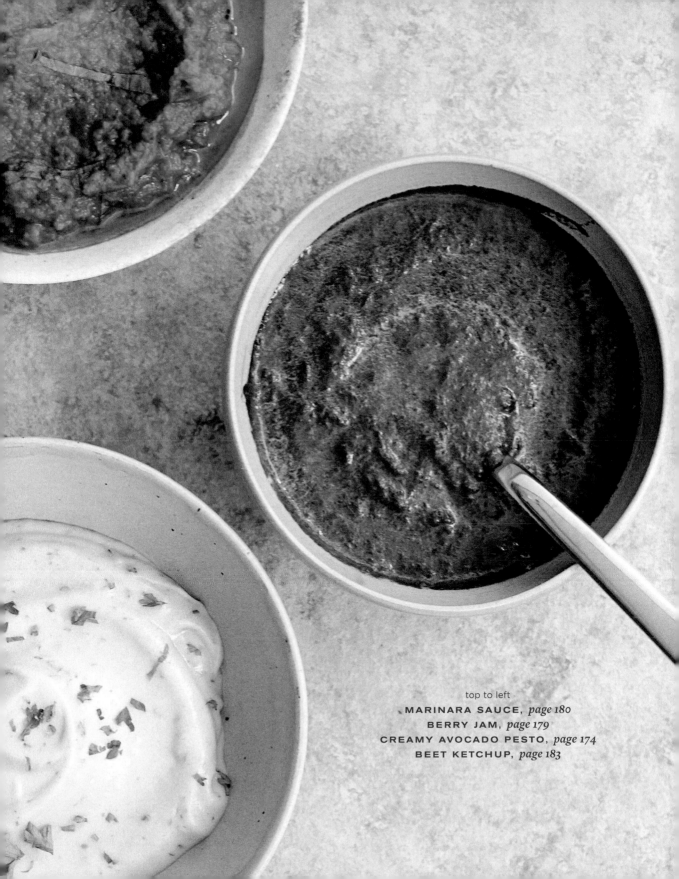

top to left
MARINARA SAUCE, *page 180*
BERRY JAM, *page 179*
CREAMY AVOCADO PESTO, *page 174*
BEET KETCHUP, *page 183*

TAHINI DRESSING

YIELDS ⅔ CUP
Prep Time: 5 to 10 minutes

½ teaspoon manuka honey
⅓ cup ice-cold filtered water, plus more as needed
⅓ cup tahini
Zest of 1 lemon
½ teaspoon ground sumac
¼ teaspoon ground cumin
1 (1-inch) piece of fresh ginger, peeled and grated
1 teaspoon soy sauce
2 tablespoons olive oil

In the Middle East and the Mediterranean region, tahini dressing is as ubiquitous as ketchup or ranch dressing is in America. Used on vegetables and meats, tahini gives any plate or sandwich that extra kick. As Acid Watchers, we are staying away from the garlic and lemon juice that flavor traditional tahini dressing, replacing these taste enhancers with a combination of soy sauce, honey, ginger, and lemon zest. Dress any salad with it, or the Pan-Seared Falafel (page 136), or serve the sauce alongside roasted winter vegetables like Brussels sprouts or beets.

In a small bowl, dilute the honey in the cold filtered water, whisking well. Add the tahini and continue whisking vigorously until the mixture is integrated and silky. Stir in the lemon zest, sumac, cumin, ginger, and soy sauce. When fully incorporated, whisk in a thin, steady stream of olive oil. Refrigerate the dressing for 30 minutes before serving. If the mixture thickens, add more water, 1 teaspoon at a time, right before serving.

GARLIC AIOLI

YIELDS ½ CUP

Prep and Cook Time: 45 minutes, plus
an overnight soak for the cashews

---

1 whole garlic head
3 teaspoons olive oil
½ cup raw unsalted cashews,
  soaked overnight
1 tablespoon lemon zest
7 tablespoons filtered water
2 teaspoons apple cider vinegar
¼ teaspoon finely ground Celtic salt

Aioli is typically made with raw garlic, raw egg, and vegetable oil. Cooking garlic significantly dampens the carminative effect of raw garlic in this healthy, egg-free aioli. The cashews that are used in this recipe neutralize the acidity of the apple cider vinegar, thus making this dip Acid Watcher–secure for the Maintenance Phase. The lemon zest, surprisingly, is not acidic.

1   Preheat the oven to 400°F.

2   To roast the garlic, cut off the top (stem end) of the garlic and peel off the outer papery layer. Place the garlic head on a square of aluminum foil and drizzle the garlic with a teaspoon of olive oil. Wrap the garlic in the foil, leaving a small opening. Bake for 35 minutes. Remove the wrapped garlic from the oven and let cool for several minutes. Unwrap the garlic and squeeze out the cloves; reserve the rest of the garlic (see Kitchen Note).

3   Drain and rinse the cashews. Place them in a blender along with the remaining 2 teaspoons olive oil, lemon zest, filtered water, vinegar, salt, and 6 cloves of the roasted garlic. Blend on high speed for 2 to 3 minutes, until completely smooth and creamy. Serve immediately. Refrigerate in an airtight container for up to 2 days.

KITCHEN NOTE   Reserve the remaining roasted garlic for other uses; add the remaining roasted garlic to a 6-ounce mason jar, submerge in olive oil, and seal. It should keep for 3 days refrigerated in an airtight container.

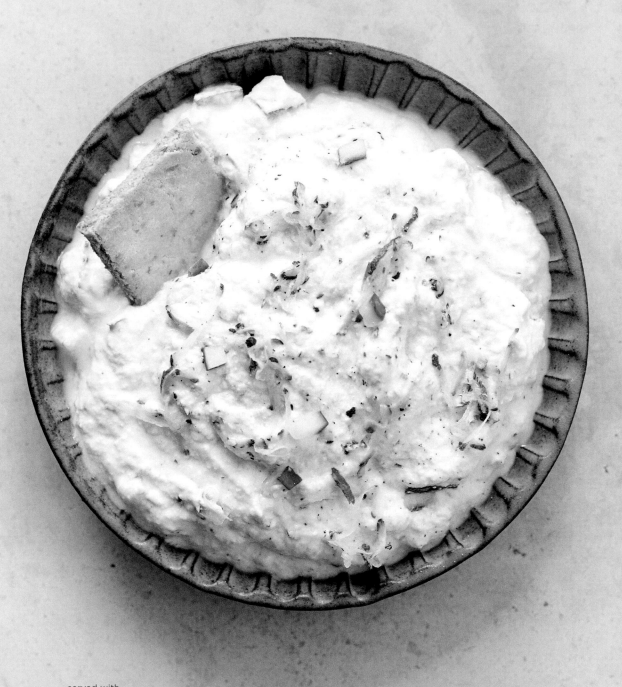

served with
**THE ACID WATCHER
CRACKER,** *page 93*

TZATZIKI SAUCE

SERVES 2

Prep Time: 10 minutes, plus an overnight soak for the cashews

---

½ cup raw unsalted cashews, soaked overnight
6 tablespoons filtered water
¾ teaspoon finely ground Celtic salt
Zest of 1 lemon
½ cup chopped English cucumber
1 tablespoon chopped fresh parsley
1 tablespoon chopped fresh cilantro

Tzatziki is generally made with raw garlic and dairy yogurt, both of which can lead to bloating, especially in combination. This Acid Watcher tzatziki is dairy- and garlic-free and is a wonderful dip for Mediterranean dishes such as the Pan-Seared Falafel (page 136) as well as for the Veggie Burgers (page 138), salmon, and turkey.

1   Rinse and drain the cashews and place them in a blender along with the filtered water, salt, and lemon zest. Blend on high speed until completely creamy, 1 to 2 minutes.

2   Add the cucumber, parsley, and cilantro. Pulse once or twice, until the cucumber is coarsely dispersed throughout and the herbs speckle the dressing. Refrigerate in an airtight container until ready to use the same day.

CREAMY AVOCADO PESTO

SERVES 2
Prep Time: 10 minutes

---

1 ripe Hass avocado, peeled
   and pitted
1 tablespoon fresh lemon juice
2 tablespoons thinly sliced
   Parmesan cheese shards
¼ teaspoon coarsely ground
   Celtic salt
½ cup baby spinach
¼ cup packed fresh basil
2½ tablespoons olive oil

Avocado and greens, both of which are alkaline, will neutralize the acidity of the lemon juice in this recipe.

1   In the bowl of a food processor, combine the avocado, lemon juice, Parmesan, salt, spinach, and basil, adding a slow, steady stream of olive oil through the feed tube while the ingredients process. Process until relatively smooth (bits of Parmesan and speckling of green from the basil and spinach will be apparent).

2   Serve this as a dip on its own or as a sauce or topping for pasta or a grain. If you're serving it with pasta, reserve a little bit of the pasta cooking water and add it to your serving bowls to thin the sauce. The pesto sauce should be served immediately at room temperature.

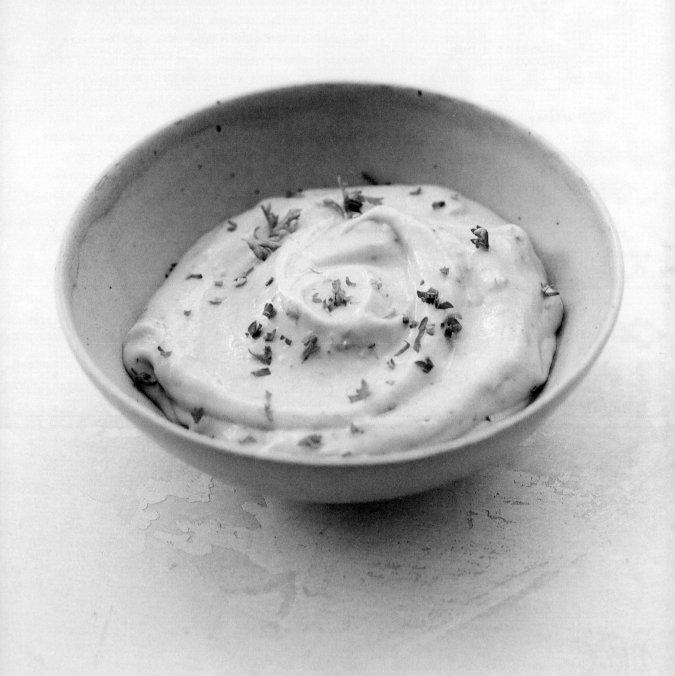

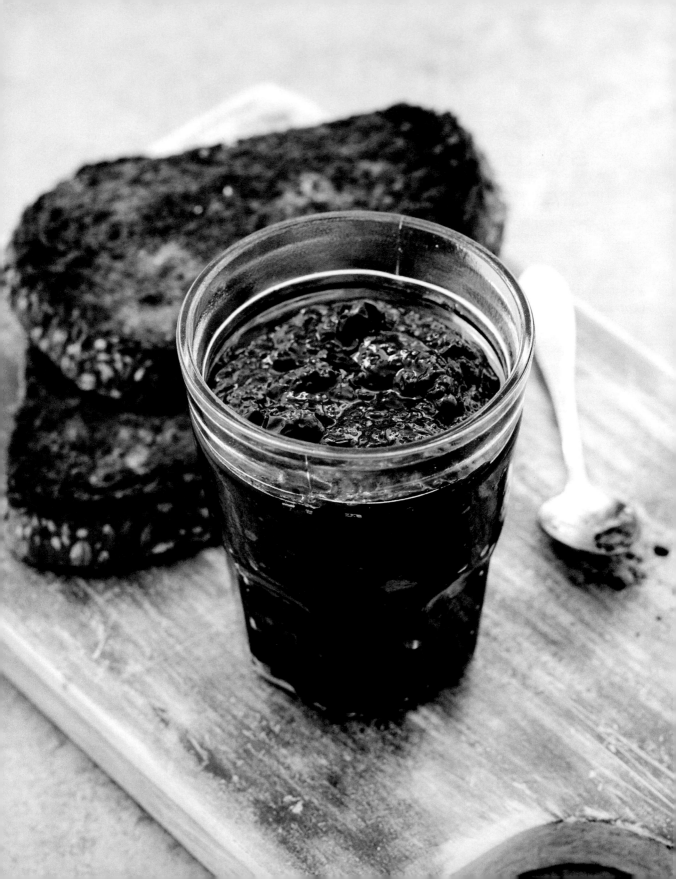

BERRY JAM

YIELDS ½ CUP
Prep and Cook Time: 10 minutes,
plus more for cooling

½ cup fresh blueberries
½ cup fresh blackberries
2 teaspoons raw honey
1 tablespoon chia seeds

Processed sugar is generally a primary ingredient of most jams and preserves. To make matters worse, especially for an Acid Watcher, the entire concoction is typically very acidic. To address these problems, we used raw honey and combined the relatively less acidic blueberries with the more acidic blackberries to create a jam above pH 4.

Unlike traditional jam filled with acid and preservatives, this mixture will last only 3 or 4 days in the fridge.

1   In a small saucepan, bring the berries and honey to a boil, stirring once to combine. Reduce the heat to low and mash the berries with a potato masher to break them down as much as possible. If, despite your efforts, some berry chunks remain, that's fine and natural. Add the chia seeds and bring the mixture to a boil. Remove from the heat and let cool for 1 minute.

2   Transfer the mixture to an airtight jar and refrigerate for at least 6 hours or up to overnight before serving. As the mixture cools, the chia seeds will absorb the excess moisture and thicken your jam!

MARINARA SAUCE

YIELDS 2¼ CUPS

Prep and Cook Time: 1 hour 5 minutes

---

2 pounds plum tomatoes
1 teaspoon olive oil
½ cup chopped carrot
¼ cup chopped celery
1½ teaspoons finely ground Celtic salt
¼ cup whole fresh basil leaves

We are very excited to present an Acid Watcher–friendly tomato sauce designed for Maintenance Phase use (foods above pH 4). We've cut out vegetables that have carminative properties, such as onion and garlic, and by adding alkaline carrot and celery, the acidity of the cooked tomatoes is relatively neutralized. This recipe, which includes fresh tomato, utilizes a technique called *concassé* to peel the tomato skin.

1   Bring a large pot of water to a boil over high heat. Fill a large bowl with ice and cold tap water and set it aside.

2   With a sharp paring knife, cut an X into the bottom of each tomato. Place the prepared tomatoes into the boiling water until the skins begin to peel back, about 25 seconds. Quickly scoop the tomatoes out of the boiling water with a slotted spoon or tongs and transfer them to the ice-water bath to stop the cooking process. After 1 to 2 minutes, peel the tomatoes.

3   Cut the tops off the tomatoes and squeeze out the juice and seeds. Strain the seeds from the tomato juice, discarding the seeds and saving the juice. Coarsely chop the tomatoes.

4   In a large saucepan over medium heat, heat the olive oil and add the carrot, celery, and ½ teaspoon of the salt. Sauté for 5 minutes, until the vegetables are softened and fragrant.

recipe continues

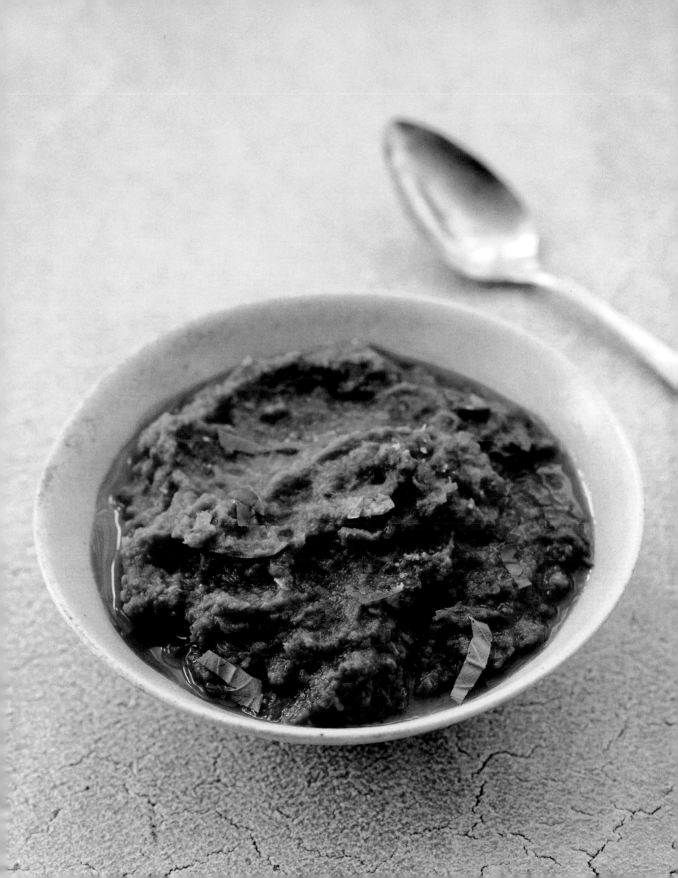

5   Add the chopped tomatoes, the reserved tomato juice, and the remaining 1 teaspoon salt to the saucepan. Cook for 5 to 10 minutes, until the tomatoes begin to break down. Crush the tomatoes with a potato masher, then stir in the fresh basil. Let simmer for 15 to 20 minutes until the sauce appears dark red and slightly thickened.

6   Remove the basil leaves and transfer the sauce to a blender. Blend until smooth, about 1 minute. Store in the refrigerator for up to 5 days or in the freezer for up to 2 months.

BEET KETCHUP

YIELDS 2 CUPS

Prep and Cook Time with raw beets:
1½ hours
Prep and Cook Time with precooked
beets: 15 minutes

4 medium raw beets (about
  14 ounces), or 2 (8.8-ounce)
  packages precooked organic beets
2 tablespoons olive oil
1 cup coarsely chopped yellow onion
1 teaspoon finely ground Celtic salt
2 tablespoons distilled white vinegar

Traditional tomato ketchup is very acidic, so we need an alternative for the Acid Watcher Diet. The problem is that ketchup generally needs vinegar, and tomatoes are not alkaline enough to neutralize the acidity of vinegar. Beets are sometimes used alongside tomato or on their own as a base for ketchup. It occurred to us that beets would likely neutralize vinegar, since they are much more alkaline and denser than tomato. How much vinegar they could neutralize was unknown. After trying different ratios of vinegar to beet, we were able to achieve the same tang and mouthfeel as traditional ketchup. Importantly, if you are using precooked organic beets, which typically come in 8.8-ounce packages, the ketchup will look pink, not "beet red." When using fresh (not precooked) beets, although the preparation is more time consuming, you will have the traditional red color of ketchup.

1 If you're using raw beets, preheat the oven to 400°F. (If you're using precooked beets, skip to the next step.) Lay a double layer of aluminum foil on a baking sheet. Place the beets on top, then wrap them into a tightly sealed bundle. Bake for 1 to 1½ hours, until a fork slides easily through the beets. Remove the beets from the oven, unwrap and let them cool slightly, then gently rub them with paper towels to remove their skins. Coarsely chop the beets and set them aside.

recipe continues

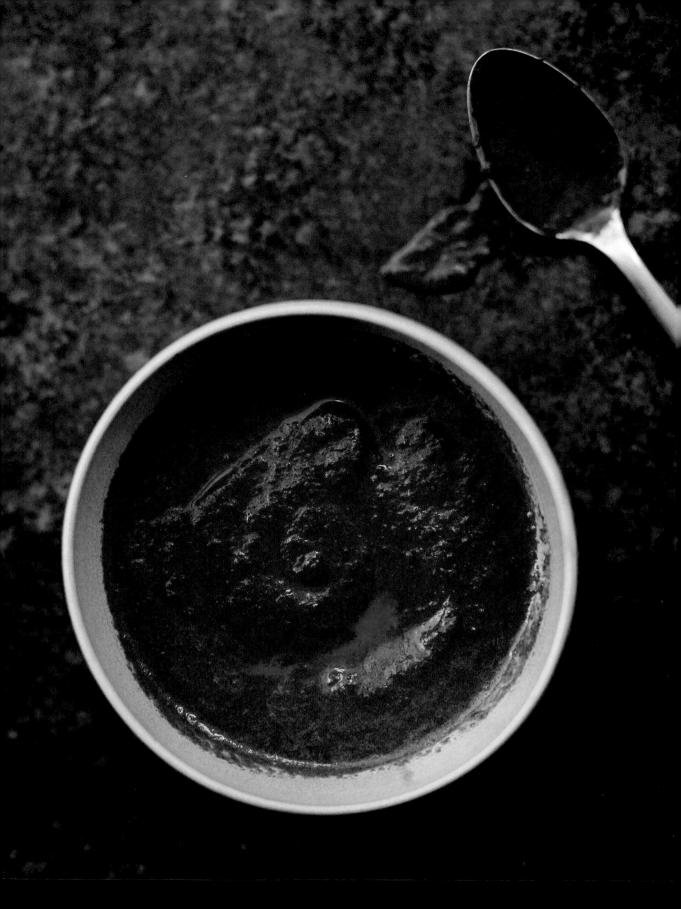

2   In a medium skillet, warm the olive oil over medium
    high heat, and add the onions and salt. Sauté for
    2 minutes, then pour in ½ cup of water. Cook for
    about 5 minutes, stirring occasionally, or until the
    water has evaporated and the onion has softened.

3   Place the cooked or precooked beets, onion, and
    vinegar into a blender and puree on high until
    completely smooth. The beet ketchup can be stored
    in an airtight container in the refrigerator for up to
    2 weeks.

NONDAIRY "MILKS"

The idea that we can make our own nondairy "milks" at home, rather than buying them already produced in stores, originally seemed daunting. So we dipped our toes in the proverbial homemade waters by starting to make almond milk at home. The concept of using a nut bag, or a nut milk bag, also initially raised eyebrows ("Where the heck are we gonna find a nut milk bag?"). It was all much ado about nothing (see the Cauliflower Pizza recipe, page 142). The main surprise was how easy it is to make nondairy milks at home. Here are the basic recipes for coconut, cashew, and almond "milks."

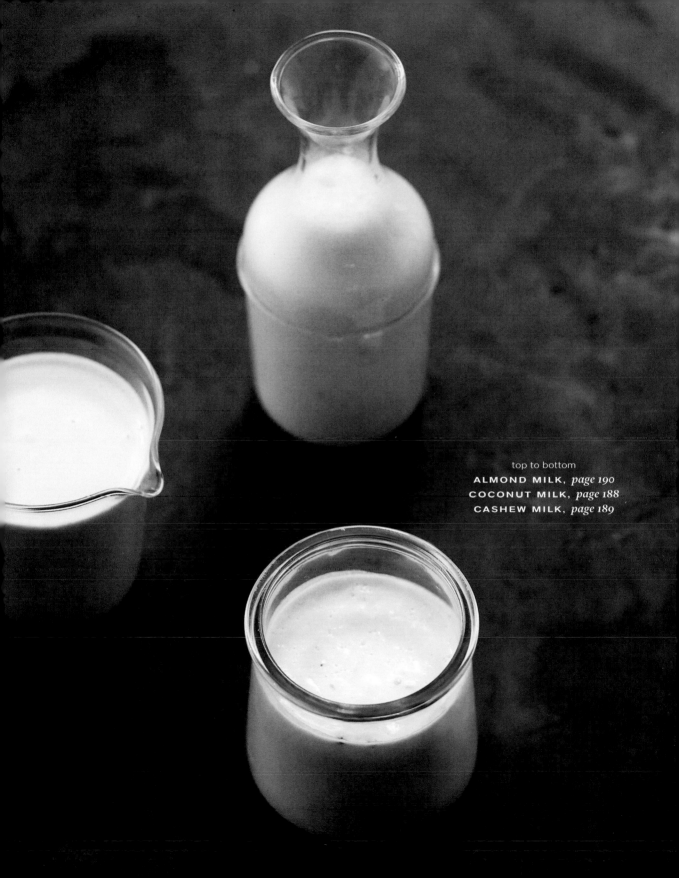

top to bottom
ALMOND MILK, *page 190*
COCONUT MILK, *page 188*
CASHEW MILK, *page 189*

COCONUT MILK

SERVES 2
Prep Time: 10 minutes

2 to 2½ cups filtered water, depending on how thick you like your coconut milk
1 cup unsweetened shredded coconut
Pinch of Celtic salt (optional)
1 Medjool date, pitted (optional)

Coconut milk is a very concentrated alkaline beverage that can readily neutralize the acidity of fruits in a smoothie. It is also delicious as an accompaniment to GrAWnola (page 72).

Place the filtered water and shredded coconut in a blender and blend on high speed for approximately 1 minute until well combined. Use 2 cups of water for thicker milk and 2½ for thinner milk. For a sweeter milk, puree the coconut and water with a pinch of Celtic salt and a Medjool date. Strain the mixture through a nut milk bag and store in the fridge for up to 3 days in an airtight container. Shake before using.

CASHEW MILK

YIELDS 6 CUPS

Prep Time: 10 minutes, plus an
overnight soak for the cashews
(we recommend at least 12 hours)

1 cup raw unsalted cashews, soaked
overnight
6 cups filtered water

The great thing about cashew milk is that it doesn't
require straining—just blend and enjoy!

Drain and rinse the soaked cashews. Combine the
cashews and filtered water in a blender and blend
on high speed until smooth, approximately 1 minute.
Pour into glasses and enjoy. Generally, this will last in
an airtight container in the refrigerator for 3 days, but
individual results may vary. Shake before using if it has
been refrigerated.

ALMOND MILK

YIELDS 5 CUPS
Prep Time: 5 minutes, plus an
overnight soak for the almonds
(we recommend 12 hours)

1 cup raw organic almonds, soaked
overnight
5 cups filtered water, plus more
as needed

Simple to make, healthier, tastier, and less costly than store-bought almond milk, homemade almond milk is now our go-to nondairy "milk."

Rinse and drain the almonds. In a blender, place the soaked almonds and filtered water using the 1:5 ratio: use 1 cup less water to make a thicker almond milk; use 1 cup more water to make a thinner almond milk. Blend on high speed for 1 minute. Pour the mixture into the nut milk bag, milking the bag as you would a cow's udder (see Note). The resulting almond milk should be refrigerated in an airtight container, where it will stay fresh for about 3 days. Shake before using after refrigeration.

NOTE Almonds are a tree nut. If you're feeling saucy, you can complete this "journey of an almond" by saving the almond pulp from the nut milk bag to make almond meal. So don't throw out the mixture in the nut milk bag; place it in the fridge, and when you are ready, dehydrate or dry the almond pulp. To do so, spread out the pulp on a baking sheet lined with parchment paper and place it in the oven at the lowest heat possible for about 3 hours. Once it is dry, let it cool. Then, process it in a food processor to get a finer texture—and you have almond meal ready for cooking. Keep the almond meal sealed in an airtight container. It stays fresh in the fridge for about 1 week.

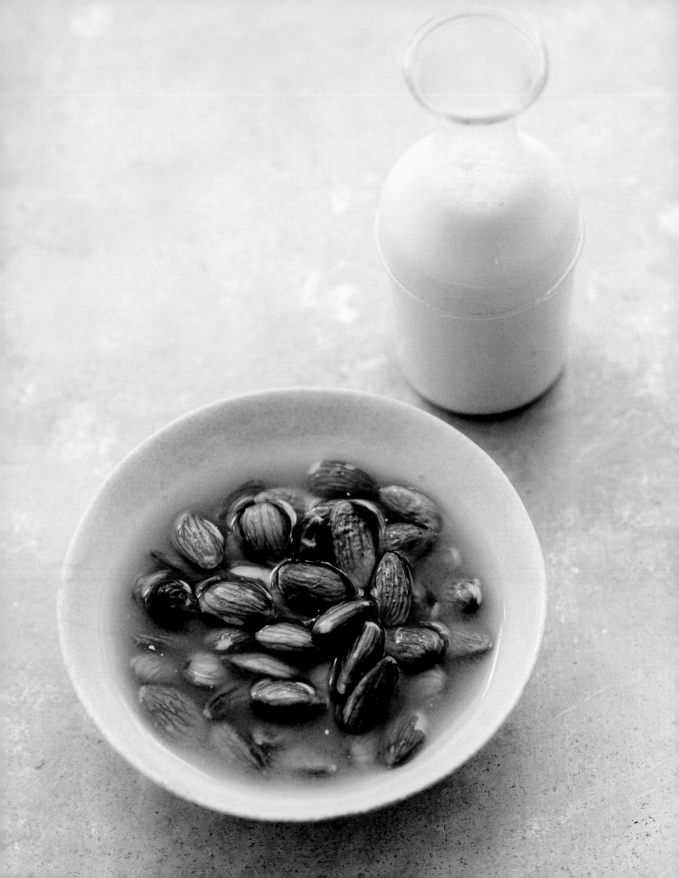

SWEETS

H HEALING PHASE   M MAINTENANCE PHASE

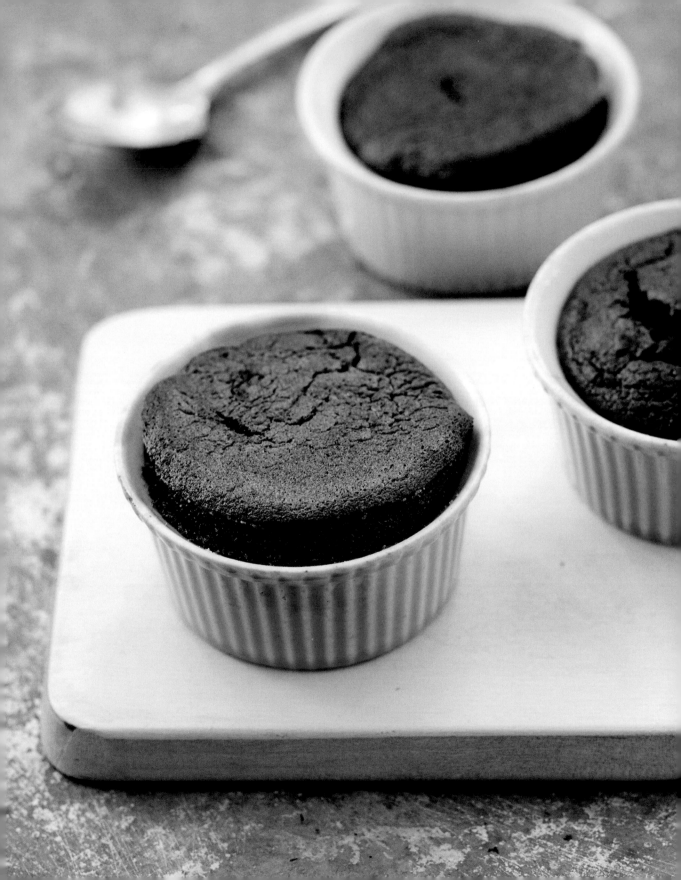

CAROB SOUFFLÉ MINIS

SERVES 5

Prep and Cook Time: 30 minutes

¼ cup coconut oil, plus more for the ramekins

½ cup carob powder

¼ cup pure maple syrup

3 large eggs, separated (see Note below)

1 teaspoon pure vanilla extract

¼ teaspoon finely ground Celtic salt

⅛ teaspoon cream of tartar

Chocolate can bother those with acid reflux, because it both loosens the lower esophageal muscle and increases acid production by the stomach. As an alternative to chocolate, without the loosening and acid-increasing side effects, we utilize carob to create this mouthwatering Acid Watcher–friendly Healing Phase treat.

1   Preheat the oven to 375°F. Position a rack in the middle of the oven. Brush five 3-inch ramekins (see Note 1) with some coconut oil. Place them on a baking sheet and set aside.

2   In a small saucepan over medium heat, combine the carob powder, ¼ cup coconut oil, maple syrup, and 2 tablespoons of water. Whisk just until smooth, about 1 minute. Transfer the carob mixture to a large bowl and let cool. Whisk in the egg yolks, vanilla, and salt. Set aside.

3   In a medium bowl, combine the egg whites and cream of tartar. Beat with a mixer on high until you reach stiff peaks, about 1 minute.

recipe continues

NOTE 1   You can use different-size ramekins, but this may affect the cooking time. Add more time for larger ramekins and less time for smaller ramekins.

NOTE 2   Crack the eggs very carefully when separating so that the yolks don't break. The egg whites won't whip properly if there is even a drop of egg yolk in them.

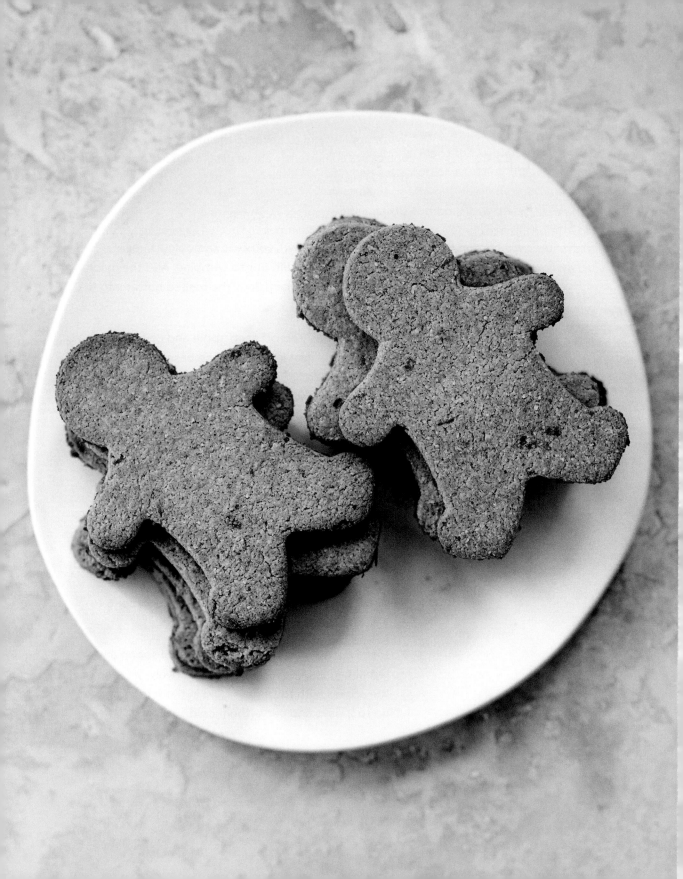

Gingerbread COOKIES

MAKES ABOUT TWELVE 4 X 3-INCH GINGERBREAD COOKIES
Prep and Cook Time:
1 hour 20 minutes, plus cooling time
(2 hours in the refrigerator)

2 Medjool dates, pitted
3 tablespoons manuka honey
¼ cup olive oil
1¾ cups almond flour
¼ cup coconut flour
½ teaspoon baking soda
3 teaspoons ground ginger
1¼ teaspoons ground cinnamon
1¼ teaspoons ground nutmeg
½ teaspoon ground cloves

Traditional gingerbread cookies contain a combination of white flour, butter, shortening, molasses, brown sugar, water, egg, and vanilla. To create the Healing Phase–friendly version, the following substitutions were made: olive oil instead of butter and shortening, dates for molasses, manuka honey for brown sugar, and almond and coconut flours in place of white flour.

1 Combine the dates, honey, olive oil, and 2 tablespoons of water in a blender and blend on high until well incorporated, approximately 1 minute. Add both flours, baking soda, and all the spices to the blender and blend on high until a dough forms. This requires you to manually work the dough between blending bursts with a rubber spatula; really get in there and make sure to scrape down all sides of the blender to incorporate as much of the wet, sticky mixture as possible. Consider the blender your mixing bowl, and don't rely on the blender to do all the work for you.

2 Transfer the dough to a large mixing bowl and continue to mix and knead it with your hands. Form the dough into a ball, cover the bowl with plastic wrap, and refrigerate for 2 hours.

3 Preheat the oven to 350°F. Line two baking sheets with parchment paper and set them aside.

4 Remove the dough from the refrigerator and place it between two pieces of parchment paper on a firm work surface. Roll out the dough until it is ¼ inch thick. Using a cookie cutter, cut out as many

recipe continues

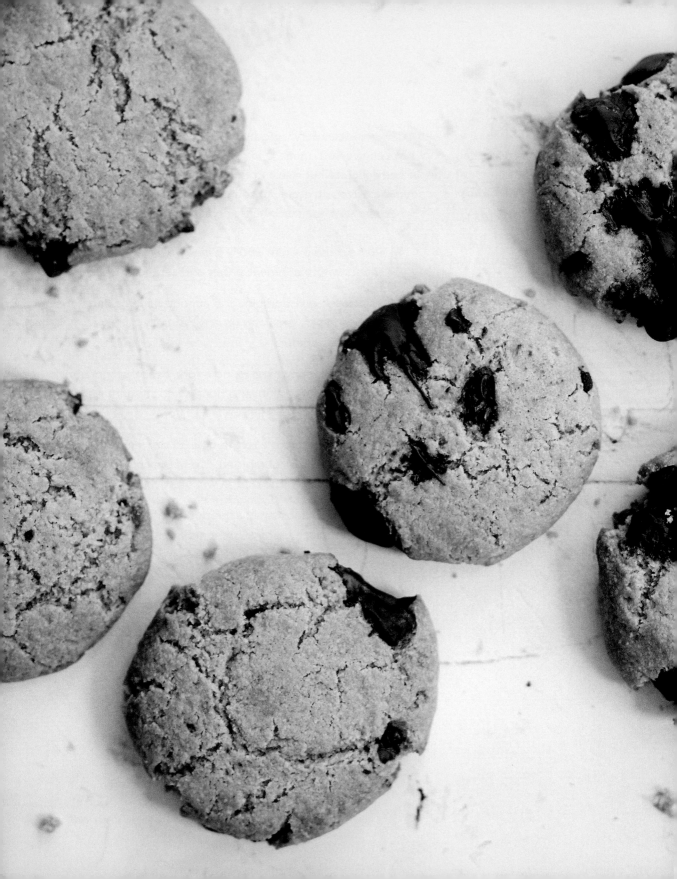

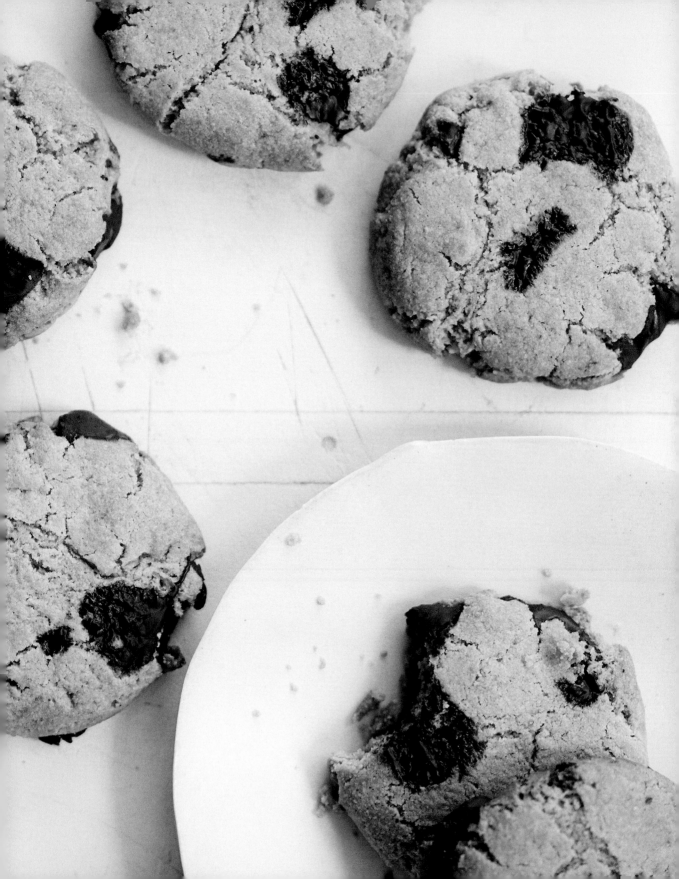

RASPBERRY COCONUT MACAROONS

MAKES 18 TO 20 MACAROONS
Prep and Cook Time: 50 minutes

1¾ cups aquafaba (from two
    15-ounce cans of chickpeas)
1 teaspoon cream of tartar
½ teaspoon coarsely ground
    Celtic salt
½ teaspoon pure vanilla extract
1 cup coconut flour
1 cup unsweetened coconut flakes
2 tablespoons pure maple syrup
¼ cup coconut oil
1 cup fresh raspberries

Aquafaba makes its appearance again (see the Real Hummus recipe, page 87) in this easy-to-make, plant-based, gluten-free Maintenance Phase treat. As previously mentioned, aquafaba is the liquid found in a can of chickpeas and, in addition to its other roles in recipes, can imitate the effects of egg whites in baking. When whipped with cream of tartar, aquafaba becomes fluffy and silky, like whipped egg whites. Make sure that the chickpeas are organic so you don't consume preservatives. Aquafaba's alkalinity helps neutralize the acidity of raspberries.

1   Preheat the oven to 350°F. Line a large baking sheet with parchment paper.

2   In a large bowl, combine the aquafaba, cream of tartar, salt, and vanilla. Using a handheld mixer with a wire whip attachment, whip the ingredients on high speed for 3 to 4 minutes, until the mixture increases in thickness and volume and soft peaks begin to form.

3   In a separate bowl, whisk the coconut flour and flakes with the maple syrup. Using a pastry cutter or a fork, mash the coconut oil into the mix until a flaky, sticky dough forms. Carefully fold in the aquafaba mix, followed by the raspberries.

4   Using a tablespoon or small ice cream scoop
    and your hands, shape the dough into small balls
    about 2 inches in diameter and place them on the
    parchment-lined baking sheet. You should have 18 to
    20 macaroons.

5   Bake the macaroons for 10 minutes, then increase
    the temperature to 400°F and bake for another 8 to
    10 minutes, until they are crispy and golden around
    the edges. Remove from the oven and allow them to
    cool completely on the baking sheet.

6   Carefully remove the fragile macaroons from the
    baking sheet using a thin wire spatula. Leftover
    cookies can be stored in an airtight container for up
    to 3 days.

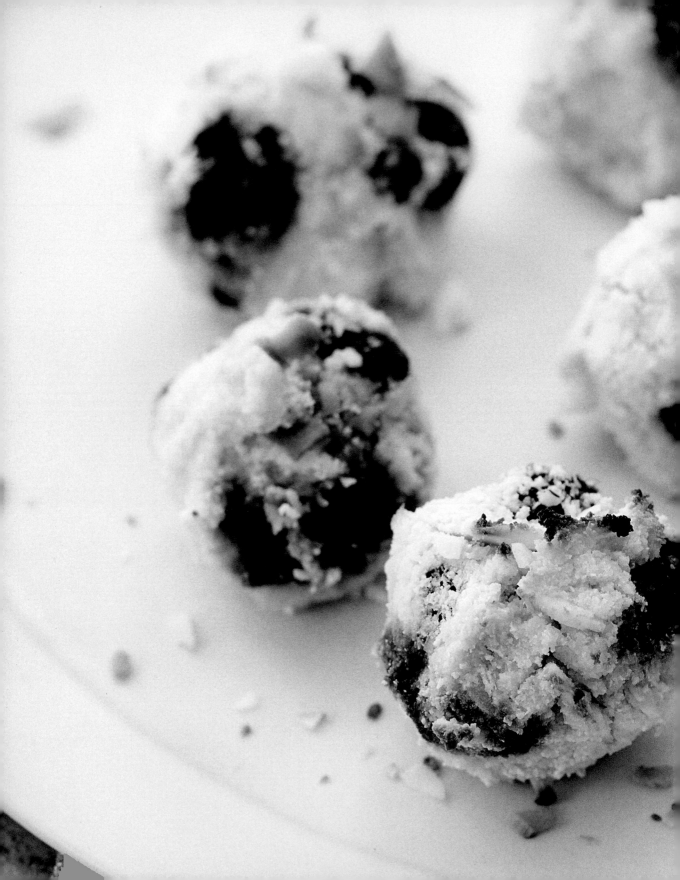

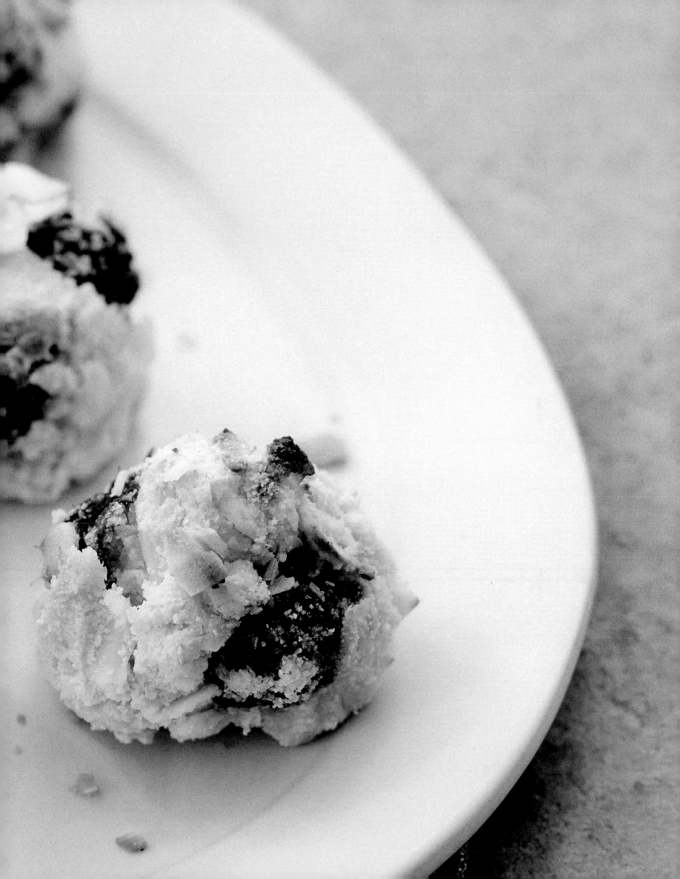

PERSIMMON BARS

MAKES 12 BARS

Prep and Cook Time: 1 hour
30 minutes, plus more for cooling

6 Fuyu persimmons
3 tablespoons pure maple syrup
1 teaspoon pure vanilla extract
¼ plus ⅛ teaspoon ground cinnamon
⅛ teaspoon ground cloves
⅓ cup coconut oil
1¾ cups almond flour, plus more
  for dusting
½ cup rye flour
2 large eggs, 1 separated
1 tablespoon olive oil, for the pan
½ cup ground pecans, ground in
  a food processor to a pebbly
  consistency

Persimmons are a late summer–early fall fruit that can be difficult to find out of season. With a pH above 5, this is a fruit to cherish on the Acid Watcher Diet. The skin of the fruit is a little dense and fibrous, which is the reason we recommend that you peel and core it—much as you would an apple or pear—for this recipe. When baked, persimmons acquire a light, candied sweetness and give these bars a jammy deliciousness. We chose Fuyu persimmons as they are not only best for baking but can also be eaten alone during the Healing Phase.

1   Peel, core, and chop the persimmons. Place them in the bowl of a food processor along with 1 tablespoon of the maple syrup, ½ teaspoon of the vanilla, ¼ teaspoon of the cinnamon, and the cloves, and pulse 4 to 5 times, until the mixture is thick but still slightly chunky, like applesauce.

2   Transfer the mixture to a heavy-bottomed saucepan over medium heat and bring it to a low boil. Continue to simmer for about 5 minutes, or until the excess liquid evaporates and the persimmon sauce thickens to a paste. Remove from the heat to cool slightly.

3   In a large bowl, combine the coconut oil, 1½ cups of the almond flour, the rye flour, 1 tablespoon of the maple syrup, 1 whole egg, and the egg yolk of the second egg (reserve the white for later). Using a pastry cutter or a fork, mash the ingredients thoroughly until the dough starts to form, turns pasty, and begins to separate from the bowl. Roll the dough into a ball, wrap in plastic wrap, and refrigerate for 30 minutes.

4   Preheat the oven to 375°F. Line a 9 × 9-inch baking pan with parchment paper. Brush the parchment paper and the sides of the baking pan with olive oil, making sure every spot is covered.

5   Remove the dough from the fridge and place it on a large cutting board dusted with 1 to 2 tablespoons of the almond flour. Using a rolling pin also lightly dusted with almond flour, roll out the dough approximately ½ inch thick. The dough will resist and fall apart, but don't worry. Whatever shape the dough is in, transfer it to the baking pan and patch and fill in the gaps with dough; it will come together and hold firmly as it bakes. Spread the persimmon paste evenly over the top of the dough leaving a border.

6   In a large bowl and using a handheld mixer, whip the reserved egg white until stiff peaks form, 2 to 3 minutes. Gently fold in the ground pecans, the remaining ¼ cup almond flour, ⅛ teaspoon cinnamon, ½ teaspoon vanilla, and 1 tablespoon maple syrup. Dollop this mixture on top of the persimmon paste at regular intervals and spread it with a knife to even out the surface; the egg white–pecan glaze will not cover the entire surface, but that's okay. You want to see the bubbly persimmon paste underneath.

7   Bake for 45 to 50 minutes, until the glaze crystallizes and the persimmon paste is glassy and amber in color. Remove from the oven and cool to room temperature. Using a sharp knife, cut 12 bars and serve. The bars will store well in an airtight container for up to 1 day.

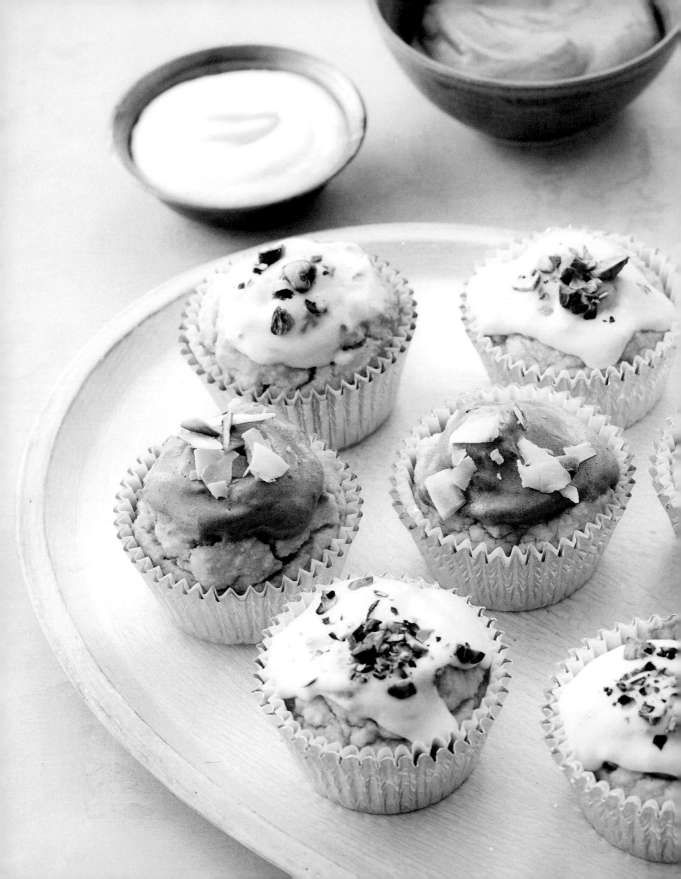

VANILLA BIRTHDAY CUPCAKES

with Vanilla and "Chocolate" Frosting

MAKES 16 CUPCAKES
Prep and Cook Time: 2 hours

FROSTING
4-ounces coconut crème
  (such as Trader Joe's)
⅛ teaspoon ground cardamom
¼ teaspoon ground cinnamon
1 tablespoon pure maple syrup
1 tablespoon carob powder

GARNISHES
2 tablespoons crumbled pistachios
2 tablespoons unsweetened coconut
  flakes

CUPCAKES
3 large eggs, at room temperature
¼ teaspoon pure vanilla extract
¼ cup pure maple syrup
½ cup plain coconut yogurt
½ cup almond milk
3 cups almond flour
¼ teaspoon coarsely ground
  Celtic salt
2 teaspoons baking powder

Just because you are an **Acid Watcher** who enjoys whole grains and dairy-free desserts doesn't mean you can't celebrate birthdays in style. These almond flour and coconut-based cupcakes are rich and flavorful without being inflammatory. With two frostings—vanilla and "chocolate"—you will have all you need for a satisfying dessert. Add another element of pizzazz on top of each cupcake with crumbled pistachios or toasted coconut flakes. Make the frosting either before the batter or while the cupcakes are baking and cooling. You'll know you've hit a recipe jackpot when the kids gobble these up.

1   **MAKE THE FROSTING:** In a medium bowl and using a handheld mixer, whip the coconut crème with the spices and maple syrup. To whip, begin on low speed (2 or 3), increase to a higher speed (4 or 5), then return back to low speed. The crème will be hard, flaky, and resistant to your efforts, but just keep going for about 5 minutes. The objective is to make the crème reach a buttery consistency, soft enough to spread on the cupcake with a knife.

2   Divide the frosting in half, placing each half in a separate bowl. Leave one half as is (vanilla), and whisk the carob powder into the other half, which will become the "chocolate" frosting. Cover the bowls with plastic wrap and refrigerate until ready to use.

3   **PREPARE THE GARNISHES:** Preheat a small nonstick pan over high heat and toast the pistachios for 2 to 3 minutes, stirring frequently to prevent burning. Place them in a small bowl. In the same nonstick pan, toast the coconut flakes for 3 to 5 minutes, or until

recipe continues

they turn golden brown, stirring frequently to prevent burning. Place them in a separate small bowl.

4 **MAKE THE CUPCAKES:** Preheat the oven to 350°F. Line two muffin tins with 16 paper liners.

5 In a large bowl, whisk the eggs, vanilla, maple syrup, coconut yogurt, and almond milk until well combined.

6 In a separate bowl, whisk the almond flour with the salt and baking powder. Combine the wet and dry ingredients thoroughly.

7 Using a spoon or a small ladle, evenly divide the batter between the liners, filling each about three-fourths full (about ¼ cup of batter). Bake for 30 to 35 minutes, until the tops of the cupcakes turn golden. Test by inserting a toothpick in the center, which should come out clean. Remove the cupcakes from the oven and allow them to cool completely on wire racks before frosting.

8 To frost the cupcakes, remove the frosting from the refrigerator and allow to soften a bit, but no longer than 10 minutes. Using a knife, "butter" each cupcake as desired, keeping in mind that the frosting is quite rich. Try to keep the frosting contained within the liner. It should look more like a ganache than a conventional whipped frosting. You should have 8 cupcakes with "chocolate" and 8 cupcakes with vanilla frosting.

9 Sprinkle the toasted pistachios on the vanilla frosting and the toasted coconut onto the chocolate frosting. Refrigerate until ready to serve.

PECAN PIE

SERVES 8 TO 10

Prep and Cook Time:
1 hour 10 minutes,
plus more for cooling

CRUST

2 tablespoons melted coconut oil,
  plus more for the pie dish
1¼ cups oat flour
¼ cup cold water

FILLING

3 large eggs
¾ cup pure maple syrup
2 tablespoons melted coconut oil
1 tablespoon pure vanilla extract
½ teaspoon finely ground Celtic salt
1½ cups pecans, coarsely chopped

This surprisingly easy-to-make Acid Watcher pecan pie notably omits two ingredients that are common to almost all other pecan pie recipes: corn syrup and vegetable shortening. Instead, we use pure maple syrup and coconut oil.

1   **MAKE THE CRUST:** Preheat the oven to 350°F. Position a rack in the middle of the oven. Lightly oil a 9-inch pie dish. In a medium bowl, combine the oat flour, coconut oil, and cold water, and mix them with your hands until they become a smooth and homogeneous dough. Press the dough evenly into the bottom of the pie dish and up the sides. Bake for 15 minutes, remove it from the oven, and set it aside.

2   **MAKE THE FILLING:** In a large bowl, beat the eggs until completely smooth. Whisk in the maple syrup, coconut oil, vanilla, and salt. Add the pecans and stir to combine. Pour the pecan mixture into the partially baked pie crust, and place in the center of the oven.

3   Bake for 45 minutes, until the filling is puffed up and slightly bubbling. Set onto a cooling rack and allow to cool for at least 1 hour before serving.

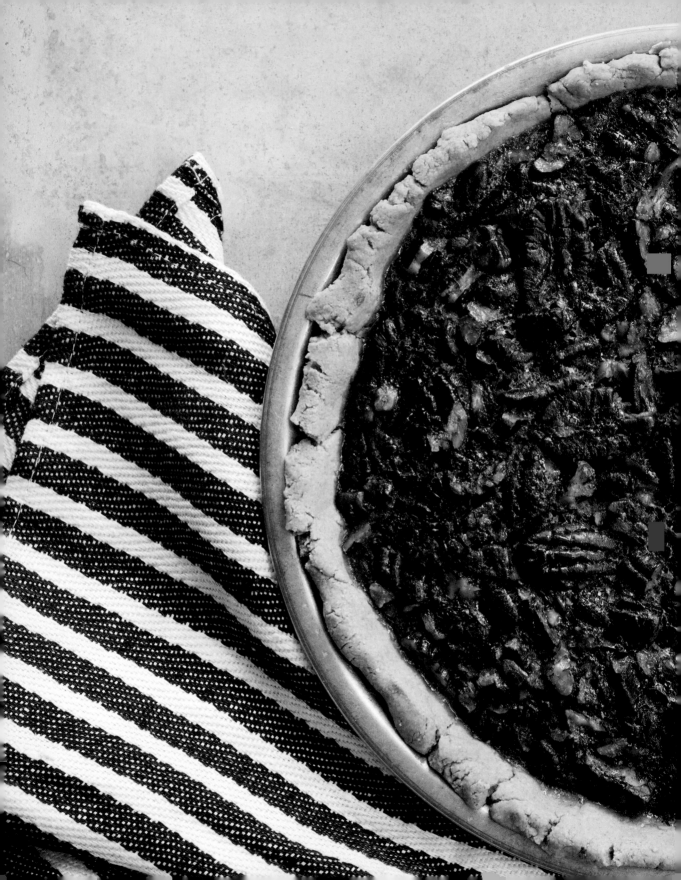

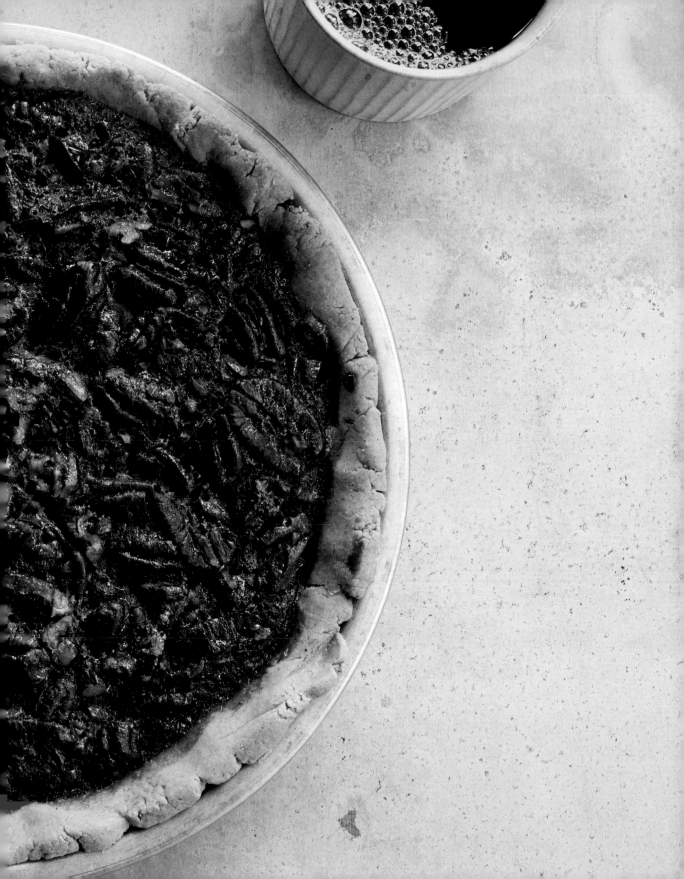

Plant-Based
EGGNOG

SERVES 2
Prep Time: 10 minutes

1½ cups almond milk
2 small ripe bananas
2 Medjool dates, pitted
½ teaspoon pure vanilla extract
¼ teaspoon ground nutmeg
¼ teaspoon ground cinnamon
1 whole clove
Pinch of Celtic salt

Eggs, sugar, milk, cream, and, voilà, eggnog! Right? Not so fast. While the pH of our "eggnAWg" is above 5, it is classified as a Maintenance Phase dish because the spices are not cooked, and their carminative properties can be troublesome for those with reflux disease. By combining spices with dates, bananas, and almond milk, a healthier and very delicious nog results.

Combine all the ingredients in a blender and blend on high speed until smooth, about 1 minute. Serve immediately.

THE ACTION PLAN

	MONDAY	TUESDAY	WEDNESDAY
BREAKFAST	KEY LIME PIE SMOOTHIE	TOFU SCRAMBLE, WATERMELON CUCUMBER JUICE	HOT QUINOA BREAKFAST PORRIDGE with BOSC PEAR
SNACK	CELTIC-SALTED KALE CHIPS	LEMON CHIA PUDDING (omit blueberries)	BEET APPLE GINGER JUICE
LUNCH	VEGGIE BURGER	WILD SALMON BURGER	KALE and BRUSSELS CAESAR SALAD
SNACK	NUT and SEED POWER BAR	THE ACID WATCHER CRACKER, with ALMOND BUTTER	PUFFED KAMUT SUNFLOWER SEED BUTTER BAR
DINNER	GLUTEN-FREE "BREADED" CHICKEN TENDERS with HEMPSEED and ALMOND FLOUR, CAESAR DRESSING, GREEN BEANS "ALMONDINE"	VEGGIE STIR-FRY in BROWN SAUCE	SESAME-CRUSTED TUNA with ZOODLES and PEANUT SAUCE

THURSDAY	FRIDAY	SATURDAY	SUNDAY
BEET BERRY SMOOTHIE	BLACK CHERRY YOGURT, WALNUTS	CREAMY HERB-INFUSED FRITTATA, WATERMELON CUCUMBER JUICE	BANANA BLENDER PANCAKES or GLUTEN-FREE OAT WAFFLES, CHICORY and VANILLA CAFFEINE-FREE LATTE
NUT and SEED POWER BAR	MISO SOUP	PUFFED KAMUT SUNFLOWER SEED BUTTER BAR	ZUCCHINI FRIES
LENTIL SOUP	SPINACH and GRILLED ASIAN PEAR SALAD with SESAME DRESSING	VEGGIE BURGER	PAN-SEARED FALAFEL, TZATZIKI SAUCE
THE ACID WATCHER CRACKER, with MACADAMIA NUT "RICOTTA"	THE ACID WATCHER CRACKER with HONEY and PEANUT BUTTER	CELTIC-SALTED KALE CHIPS	CHAWCOLATE HAZELNUT SHAKE
COCONUT SHRIMP, SWEET POTATO MASH	ACID WATCHER EGGS BENEDICT (aka GREEN EGGS WITHOUT HAM)	GRILLED SALMON with CRISPY SKIN, STEAMED ASPARAGUS with SHAVED PARMESAN	ED'S SUNDAY NIGHT WHOLE ROAST CHICKEN, BAKED CARROTS

	MONDAY	TUESDAY	WEDNESDAY
BREAKFAST	ORANGE CREAM SMOOTHIE	LEMON BLUEBERRY CHIA PUDDING	CINNAMON RAISIN GRAWNOLA, NONDAIRY MILK
SNACK	REAL! GUACAMOLE, VEGGIES	REAL HUMMUS, VEGGIES	TEXTURE and COLOR RIOT TRAIL MIX
LUNCH	BEET SALAD with MACADAMIA NUT "RICOTTA" and MANGO "VINAIGRETTE"	APPLE, FENNEL, and ARUGULA SALAD	TOFU WALDORF SALAD
SNACK	THE ACID WATCHER CRACKER with BERRY JAM	NUT and SEED POWER BAR	MAGRA'S BABA (BABA GHANOUJ)
DINNER	TURKEY MEATBALLS, MARINARA SAUCE	GRILLED FISH TACOS	CAULIFLOWER "FRIED" RICE

THURSDAY	FRIDAY	SATURDAY	SUNDAY
PUMPKIN PIE SMOOTHIE	MEDITERRANEAN BANANA BREAD, CHICORY and VANILLA CAFFEINE-FREE LATTE	HUEVOS RANCHEROS	CINNAMON RAISIN FRENCH TOAST
BAKED CORN TORTILLA CHIPS, PICO DE GALLO	PUFFED KAMUT SUNFLOWER SEED BUTTER BAR	APPLE and PEAR SAUCE	NUT and SEED POWER BAR
GREEK SALAD with CHICKPEAS	SPLIT PEA SOUP	TOMATO BASIL SOUP	QUINOA TABBOULEH
FRESH PEA VICHYSSOISE	THE ACID WATCHER CRACKER, CHOPPED "LIVER"	PUFFED KAMUT SUNFLOWER SEED BUTTER BAR	BLACK CHERRY YOGURT
BUTTERNUT SQUASH "MAC 'N' CHEESE"	PLANT-BASED CHILI	CAULIFLOWER PIZZA	MEDITERRANEAN MONKFISH with OLIVES, ARTICHOKES with GARLIC AIOLI

RAW FRUIT

1 Fuji apple
4 small Hass avocados
2 avocados
1 bunch medium ripe
   bananas (6 -7)
1 (6-ounce) container organic
   blackberries
10 lemons
6 limes
1 Asian pear
1 Bosc pear
1 (6-ounce) container organic
   raspberries
1 baby seedless watermelon

DRIED FRUIT

1 (8-ounce) package dried Turkish
   apricots
1 (12-ounce) bag unsweetened
   coconut flakes
1 (12-ounce) bag unsweetened
   shredded coconut
4 (6-ounce) bags pitted Deglet
   dates
1 (15-ounce) bag Medjool dates

FROZEN FRUIT

1 (10-ounce) bag frozen organic
   dark sweet cherries

PLANT PROTEIN

2 (14-ounce) blocks firm tofu
1 (14-ounce) block tofu (soft or
   firm)

VEGETABLES and HERBS

1 bunch asparagus (12 spears)
1 small package fresh bay leaves
1 pound green beans
1 pound raw beets
1 head Boston lettuce
1 pound broccoli florets
1 pound Brussels sprouts
3 pounds carrots
2 pounds cauliflower florets
3 bunches celery
1 pound dried chicory
2 bunches fresh cilantro
5 English cucumbers
2 bunches fresh dill
2 medium to large pieces fresh
   ginger
7 bunches curly kale
2 bunches lacinato or purple kale
2 (8-ounce) packages button
   mushrooms
2 large bunches fresh parsley
2 parsnips
1 small package fresh rosemary
2 pounds baby spinach
2 medium sweet potatoes
1 (2-ounce) bag wakame
1 (16-ounce) package green
   zucchini zoodles
2 medium zucchini

DRIED and CANNED LEGUMES

1 (1-pound) bag carob powder
1 (1-pound) bag dried chickpeas
1 (1-pound) bag green lentils

DRIED SPICES and HERBS

1 (2-ounce) bottle ground
   cinnamon
1 (1.4-ounce) bottle ground
   coriander
1 (2-ounce) bottle ground cumin
1 (1.48-ounce) bottle ground
   fennel seed
1 (4-ounce) bottle Mexican
   oregano
1 (1.9-ounce) bottle sweet paprika
1 (2-ounce) bottle ground sumac
1 (2-ounce) bottle ground
   turmeric

EGGS

4 dozen large organic eggs

POULTRY

12 ounces boneless skinless
   chicken breasts
1 (3½- to 4-pound) air-chilled
   fresh organic chicken

FISH AND SHELLFISH

1½ pounds skinless wild Alaskan
   salmon fillets
2 (6-ounce) skin-on wild salmon
   fillets
1 pound smoked salmon
1 pound (20 medium) wild
   shrimp, cleaned
2 (6-ounce) wild tuna steaks

NUTS and SEEDS

1 pound raw organic almonds

1 (14-ounce) bag flax seeds

2 pounds raw unsalted cashews

1 (15-ounce) bag chia seeds

1 (10-ounce) bag raw sliced
almonds

1 (1-pound) bag flaxseed meal

1 pound raw shelled hazelnuts

1 (8-ounce) bag shelled raw
hempseeds

1 pound raw unsalted macadamia
nuts

1 (2-ounce) bottle black sesame
seeds

1 (1.37-ounce) bottle toasted
sesame seeds

1 (2.2-ounce) bottle white sesame
seeds

1 (1-pound) bag raw sunflower
seeds

1 pound shelled raw walnuts

SPREADS

1 (16-ounce) jar raw organic
almond butter

1 (16-ounce) jar organic peanut
butter, smooth

1 (16-ounce) jar unsweetened
organic sunflower seed butter

1 (10.6-ounce) jar organic tahini

DAIRY

1 (16-ounce) package
(four 4-ounce sticks)
organic butter, unsalted

4 ounces Parmesan cheese

CONDIMENTS

1 (14-ounce) jar organic virgin,
unrefined coconut oil

1 (8-ounce) jar raw local honey

1 (500-gram) jar manuka honey

1 (8-ounce) bottle organic maple
syrup, Grade A, Amber Color

1 (16-ounce) container white miso

1 (16.9-ounce) bottle extra-virgin
olive oil

1 (1-pound) bag coarsely ground
Celtic salt

1 (1-pound) bag finely ground
Celtic salt

1 (10-ounce) bottle soy sauce

1 (20-ounce) bottle tamari

1 (4-ounce) bottle pure vanilla
extract

1 (16-ounce) bottle apple cider
vinegar

1 (32-ounce) bottle distilled white
vinegar

DAIRY ALTERNATIVES

2 (28-ounce) bottles
unsweetened plain almond
milk

1 (16-ounce) container
unsweetened plain coconut
milk yogurt

5 (32-ounce) containers plain
unsweetened soy milk

BREADS and GRAINS

2 (24-ounce) loaves Ezekiel
Sprouted Whole Grain bread

1 (6-ounce) bag organic puffed
Kamut cereal

1 (1-pound) bag oat flour

1 (32-ounce) bag old-fashioned
rolled oats

1 (1-pound) bag white quinoa

1 (2-pound) bag brown rice

1 (6-ounce) bag puffed brown
rice cereal

1 (8-ounce) bag unprocessed
wheat bran

GLUTEN-FREE FLOURS

1 (1-pound) bag almond flour

1 (2-pound) bag masa harina

BEVERAGES

1 case bottled water

MISCELLANEOUS

1 (10-ounce) container baking
powder

1 (16-ounce) box baking soda

RAW FRUIT

3 Gala apples

2 Golden Delicious apples

1 (16-ounce) jar unsweetened fresh applesauce

2 avocados

4 Hass avocados

1 bunch medium ripe bananas (6 to 7)

2 (6-ounce) containers organic blackberries

3 (6-ounce) containers organic blueberries

10 lemons

12 limes

2 mangoes

1 pound pitted kalamata olives

2 navel oranges

2 small papayas

2 Bosc pears

1 (10-ounce) box organic pumpkin puree

2 tangerines

DRIED FRUIT

½ pound dehydrated apples

1 pound dried Turkish apricots

1 (12-ounce) bag unsweetened coconut flakes

4 (6-ounce) bags pitted Deglet dates

1 (15-ounce) bag Medjool dates

1 pound dark raisins

PLANT PROTEIN

1 (8-ounce) block tempeh

1 (14-ounce) block firm tofu

FROZEN FRUIT

1 (10-ounce) bag frozen organic dark sweet cherries

VEGETABLES and HERBS

2 artichokes

1 pound arugula

2 large bunches fresh basil

1 small package fresh bay leaves

1 pound raw beets

6 bell peppers

1 butternut squash

1 head red cabbage

1 head white cabbage

3 pounds carrots

2 pounds riced cauliflower or 2 heads of cauliflower

3 bunches celery

2 small celery roots

1 pound dried chicory

2 bunches fresh cilantro

1 ear sweet yellow corn (omit if using frozen corn)

2 English cucumbers

1 bunch fresh dill

1 medium eggplant

2 bulbs fennel

1 head garlic

2 large pieces fresh ginger

2 jicamas

1 bunch leeks

2 medium portobello mushrooms

1 sweet onion

4 white onions

1 yellow onion

2 large bunches fresh parsley

3 parsnips

4 ounces pea shoots

4 ounces roasted peas

28 ounces fresh sweet peas (omit if using frozen peas)

1 pound romaine lettuce hearts

1 small package fresh rosemary

2 rutabagas

2 pounds baby spinach

1 small package fresh thyme

5 beefsteak tomatoes

4 (12-ounce) containers grape tomatoes

4 pounds plum tomatoes

2 turnips

FROZEN VEGETABLES

1 (10-ounce) bag sweet corn (omit if using fresh corn)

2 (14.4-ounce) bags sweet peas (omit if using fresh peas)

DRIED SPICES and HERBS

1 (3.75-ounce) bottle asafetida

1 (2-ounce) bottle ground cinnamon

1 (1.8-ounce) bottle ground cloves

1 (1.4-ounce) bottle ground coriander

1 (2-ounce) bottle ground cumin

1 (1.48-ounce) bottle ground fennel seed

1 (0.85-ounce) bottle herbes de Provence

1 (1.9-ounce) bottle ground nutmeg

1 (1.9-ounce) bottle sweet paprika

1 (2-ounce) bottle ground sumac

1 (0.5-ounce) bottle dried thyme

1 (2-ounce) bottle ground turmeric

1 (1.4-ounce) bottle za'atar

EGGS

2 dozen large organic eggs

POULTRY

2 pounds ground organic turkey

FISH and SHELLFISH

2 (6-ounce) monkfish fillets

12 ounces tilapia

NUTS and SEEDS

3 pounds raw organic almonds

3 pounds raw unsalted cashews

1 (15-ounce) bag chia seeds

1 (1-pound) bag flaxseed meal

1 (14-ounce) bag flaxseeds

1 pound unsalted raw
    macadamia nuts

1 pound shelled pistachios

1 pound raw shelled pumpkin
    seeds

1 pound raw sunflower seeds

1 pound raw shelled walnuts

GLUTEN-FREE FLOURS

1 (1-pound) bag almond flour

1 (14-ounce) bag almond meal

DAIRY ALTERNATIVES

2 (28-ounce) bottles plain,
    unsweetened almond milk

1 (16-ounce) container plain,
    unsweetened coconut milk
    yogurt

2 (32-ounce) containers plain,
    unsweetened soy milk

CONDIMENTS

1 (2.3-ounce) bottle capers in salt

1 (14-ounce) jar organic virgin,
    unrefined coconut oil

1 (8-ounce) jar raw local honey

1 (500-gram) jar manuka honey

1 (8-ounce) bottle organic maple
    syrup, Grade A, Amber Color

1 (12-ounce) jar Primal Kitchen
    eggless mayonnaise

1 (7.5-ounce) bottle Dijon mustard

1 (16.9-ounce) bottle extra-virgin
    olive oil

1 (1-pound) bag coarsely ground
    Celtic salt

1 (1-pound) bag finely ground
    Celtic salt

1 (10-ounce) bottle soy sauce

1 (4-ounce) bottle pure vanilla
    extract

1 (16-ounce) bottle apple cider
    vinegar

1 (32-ounce) bottle distilled white
    vinegar

CHEESE

4 ounces feta cheese

6 ounces Parmesan cheese

DRIED and CANNED LEGUMES

2 (15-ounce) cans organic black
    beans

1 (1-pound) bag dried chickpeas
    (omit if using canned)

2 (15-ounce) cans organic
    chickpeas (reduce to 1 can if
    using dried)

1 (1-pound) bag split peas

BREADS and GRAINS

1 (24-ounce) loaf Ezekiel 4:9
    Cinnamon Raisin Bread

1 (22-ounce) loaf whole-grain
    bread, Bread Alone Certified
    Organic Nine Mixed Grain

1 (6-ounce) bag organic puffed
    Kamut cereal

1 (8-ounce) box gluten-free elbow
    macaroni, preferably Ancient
    Harvest Gluten Free

1 (32-ounce) bag old-fashioned
    rolled oats

1 (1-pound) bag white quinoa

1 (2-pound) bag brown rice

2 (12-ounce) packages corn
    tortillas, preferably Trader
    Joe's Corn Tortillas or Ezekiel
    4:9 Sprouted Corn Tortillas

1 (8-ounce) bag unprocessed
    wheat bran

1 (5-pound) bag whole-wheat
    flour

SPREADS

1 (16-ounce) jar organic
    unsweetened sunflower seed
    butter

1 (10.6-ounce) jar organic tahini

BEVERAGES

1 case bottled water

MISCELLANEOUS

1 (10-ounce) container baking
    powder

1 (16-ounce) box baking soda

SEASONAL MENUS

Feeding and entertaining large groups of people is something entirely possible while following the Acid Watcher Diet principles, especially in the Maintenance Phase, where there are even more options.

JULY 4 BBQ

KALE AND BRUSSELS CAESAR SALAD (page 129)

QUINOA TABBOULEH (page 127)

REAL! GUACAMOLE (page 84) and BAKED CORN TORTILLA CHIPS (page 92)

VEGGIE BURGER (page 138)

WILD SALMON BURGER (page 156)

OPEN SESAME COOKIES (TAHINI COOKIES) with dark chocolate chunks (page 201)

Have a bunch of people over to enjoy the outdoors with a lighter menu that is refreshing, broadly appealing, and speaks to vegetarians and meat-eating folks alike. In particular, the cashew-based Caesar Dressing handles the sun better than traditional Caesar dressings containing raw egg and cheese.

THANKSGIVING

SWEET POTATO MASH (page 100)

BAKED CARROTS (page 96)

ED'S SUNDAY NIGHT WHOLE ROAST CHICKEN (page 160)

MUSHROOM DRESSING (page 97)

PECAN PIE (page 215)

BAKED APPLES (page 197)

Stuff your chicken with our high-fiber mushroom dressing with its powerful and traditional Thanksgiving herbal flavors (like rosemary); you won't miss the processed, nutritionally void bread-based stuffing laden with butter. We kept the traditional Thanksgiving veggies and desserts, but with a less inflammatory spin while still preserving the Fall flavors.

CHRISTMAS

APPLE, FENNEL, AND ARUGULA SALAD (page 131)

GREEN BEANS "ALMONDINE" (page 101)

GRILLED SALMON WITH CRISPY SKIN (page 137)

GINGERBREAD COOKIES (page 199)

PLANT-BASED EGGNOG (page 218)

Skip the ham and fatty roasts for this festive healthy-fat fish. Traditional, delicious, and hearty veggie sides with winter fruit and seasonal elements merge with traditional Christmas desserts to complete this Acid Watcher–friendly feast. You can even take a crack at building your own gingerbread house with our dough, gluing the gingerbread pieces together with pureed dates!

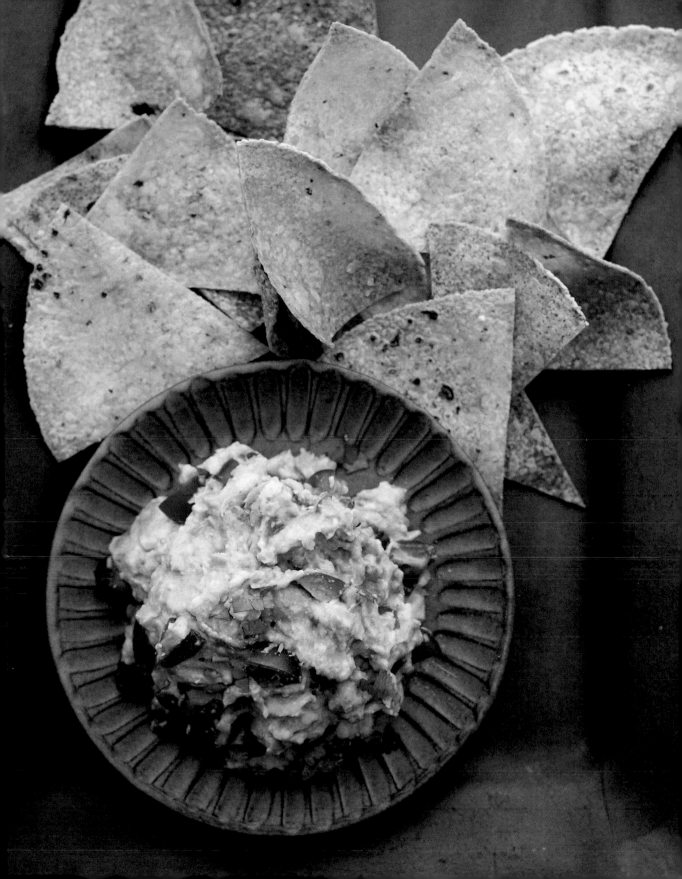

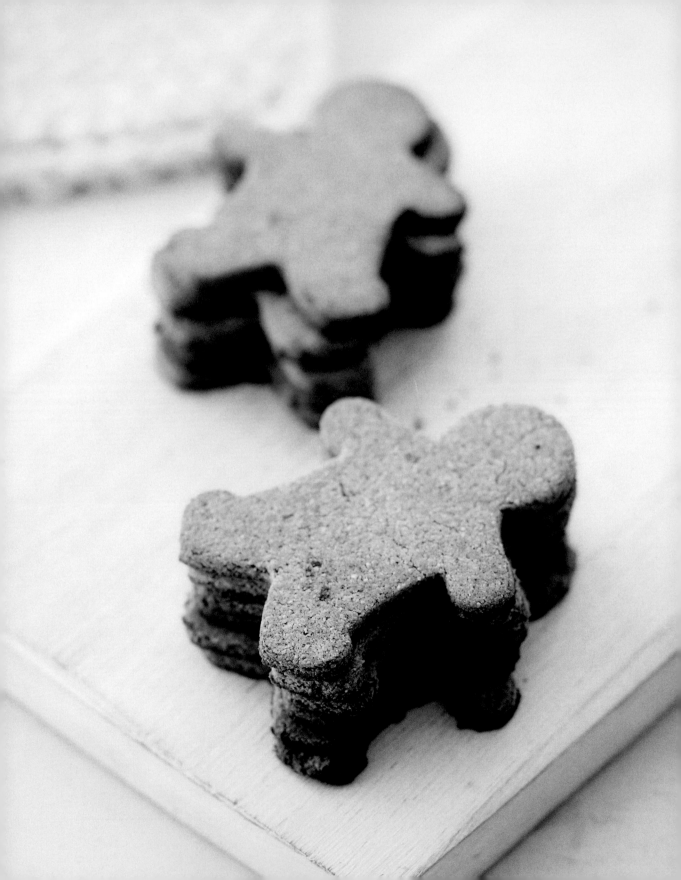

ACKNOWLEDGMENTS

Since the publication of *The Acid Watcher Diet,* I have been pushing the envelope of "food is medicine," and I would like to thank several people who have been instrumental in assisting me in creating a state-of-the-art low-acid, high-fiber diet that is anti-inflammatory for everybody.

First, thank you to my spouse and coauthor, Samara Kaufmann Aviv, who has utilized her firsthand, humbling experience with acid reflux disease as the inspiration to find a food solution to this pervasive problem. Combining her science background with cooking skills she acquired in childhood from her late mother, Samara was uniquely positioned to take the original Acid Watcher concepts expressed by Bobby Elijah Aviv and Giordana Aviv into new territory. In addition, I am exceptionally grateful to Lyzcela "Momo" Grimes, who started and continues to maintain and harness the energy of the Acid Watcher Diet Support Group and Recipe Share on Facebook. I am particularly honored to be working with the past and present moderators of this group.

Thank you to my literary agent, Steve Troha from Folio Lit, who has guided me in the development of this cookbook as well as fostering a salon of experts in the wellness space, both from the food and the fitness perspectives. Particular gratitude to chefs Julia Serebrinsky and Emiko Shimojo, who, working with Samara, have developed a reliable platform for the discovery, creation, and execution of Acid Watcher–friendly foods of all varieties. I am grateful to Diana Baroni, Michele Eniclerico, Christina Foxley, and Tammy Blake from Penguin Random House, who were instrumental in the editing and marketing of the book. I'm grateful to, and in awe of, my food photographer, Robert Bredvad, and the food styling, prop, and design team of Corey Belle,

Saori Hashimoto, Maeve Sheridan, Ashleigh Sarbone, and Sonia Persad.

Many thanks go to my professional colleagues from my years at Columbia University: Drs. Andrew Blitzer, James Dillard, J. P. Mohr, Byron Thomashow, Lanny Close, Hector Rodriguez, Joseph Haddad, Michael Sisti, Jeffrey Bruce, Ian Storper, Herbert Pardes, and Steven Corwin, and to my medical school classmate, my personal physician, and dear friend, the late Henry Lodge. I laud Florence and Herbert Irving for their largesse and vision, which enabled some of my original clinical research to be funded and carried out.

Much appreciation goes to Thomas Murry, SLP, PhD, the renowned speech-language pathologist who worked with me, side by side, for ten years at the Voice and Swallowing Center at Columbia University. In addition, speech-language pathologists Andie Schneider, Christie Block, Amanda Hembree, Eric Blicker, Manderly Cohen, Mark Berlin, Carolyn Gartner, Winston Cheng, and Marta Kazandjian have continued to be extremely helpful in the care of our patients. I'm also very thankful to registered dieticians Diane Insolia and Tanya Zuckerbrot for their wonderful care of our patients.

A special acknowledgment to Drs. Steven Zeitels, Robert Sataloff, Robert Ossoff, Stanley Shapshay, Jamie Koufman, Marshall Strome, Peter Belafsky, Greg Postma, Blake Simpson, Craig Zalvan, Charles Ford, Jeffrey Rosenbloom, and Jeffrey Gallups, who were extraordinarily supportive of using "food as medicine" to treat reflux disease, backing dietary concepts long before we had the scientific results we now know.

I would like to thank all my colleagues, staff, and administration at ENT and Allergy Associates, LLP—in particular, my fellow laryngologists at the Voice and Swallowing Center, Drs. David Godin, Joel Portnoy,

Jared Wasserman, Farhad Chowdhury, Ajay Chitkara, Philip Passalaqua, Anju Patel, Joseph Depietro, Amit Patel, Anna Stern, Chandra Ivey, and Melin Tan-Geller, who have been instrumental in helping to broaden the breadth and depth of our Voice and Swallowing Center. I would also like to thank my partners in my clinical offices: Drs. Jason Abramowitz, Sujana Chandrasekhar, Ofer Jacobowitz, Jamie Kiehm, Jason Moche, Robert Green, Steven Sachs, Scott Markowitz, Guy Lin, Won Choe, Michael Bergstein, Jill Zeitlin, John County, and Lynelle Granady. Also, special thanks to Drs. Marc Levine, Moshe Ephrat, Lee Shangold, Krzysztof Nowak, Lauren Zaretsky, and Adrianna Hekiert. I extend further expression of appreciation to my medical assistants, Cosette Osmani and Charleen Male. The administrative team at ENT and Allergy Associates, in particular Robert Glazer, Richard Effman, Jason Campbell, Nicole Monti, Drew Franklin, Rick Keifer, Jessica Rodriguez, Rosaly Hernandez, and Arthur Schwacke, were very helpful and encouraging.

Much gratitude to my medical colleagues around the country for their support: Drs. James D'Orta, Dana Thompson, Michael Benninger, Seth Dailey, David Posner, Ken Altman, Eric Genden, Peak Woo, Mark Courey, Brett Miles, Michael Goldberg, Roger Crumley, Michael Pitman, Blair Jobe, and John Hunter.

The awareness of acid reflux disease and its complications overseas was greatly enhanced by Drs. Jean Abitbol, Gabriel Jaume, Manolo Tomas, Carmen Gorriz, Lance Maron, Sarmed Sami, Krish Ragunath, and Peter Friedland.

I would like to thank the following gastroenterologists for their support and guidance: Drs. Charles Lightdale, Lawrence Johnson, Babak Mohajer, Michael Glick, Veronika Dubrovskya, David Markowitz, Jonathan LaPook, Stanley Benjamin, Phil Katz, Julian Abrams, Mark Pochapin, Arnon Lambroza, Joel Richter, Lawrence Cohen, Reza Shaker, Alin Botoman, Michael Vaezi, Greg Haber, Robert Fath, Christopher DiMaio, David Greenwald, Gina Sam, Felice Schnoll-Sussman, Sharmila Anandasabapathy, Mark Noar, Nicholas Shaheen, David Katzka, Amitabh Chak, and Ashley Faulx.

Several leaders from the medical device, pharmaceutical, and food industries were critical in the transformation of my ideas into reality, notably Lewis Pell, Katsumi Oneda, Nicholas Tsaclas, Ron Hadani, Mark Fletcher, Janis Saunier, David Damm, Ted Phelan, Alex Gorsky, Dr. Harlan Weisman, Greg Grossman, Ross Franklin, Bo Reilly, and Damion Michaels.

I am grateful to my friends and colleagues in the media and entertainment world who have brought attention to the dangers of untreated acid reflux, including Dr. Mehmet Oz, Steve Kroft, Craig Kallman, Diane Sawyer, Tracy Anderson, Kristina Bucaram, Vani Hari, Tim Sullivan, Dr. Michael Crupain, Jane Derenowski, Jane Brody, Rosanna Scotto, Carol Brodie, Ian Axel, Alex Newell, Gad Elmaleh, Jen Kirkman, Dan Soder, Gayle King, John Turturro, Aviva Drescher, DJ Camilo, Megan Ryte, and Jack Rosenthal.

Thank you to my close friends Jonathan Rapillo, Cherish Gallant, Robert Berman, Ira Kaufman, Herb Subin, Paul Michael Weiner, Jonathan Halpern, Jonathan Lowenberg, and Daniel Liebovici for their unwavering reassurance as this project developed and unfolded. I am also grateful to Samara's dear friends and colleagues Gabrielle Sholes, Brenda Maldonado, Jill Goldsmith, Kira Markowitz, Chloe Foreht, Tasha and Matthew Shields, Helene Resnick, and Brandon Perlman for their constant encouragement.

My appreciation and gratitude to Harvey Shapiro for his excellent legal advice as well as his continued friendship over the years.

A special thanks to my brother Oren Aviv and to my father-in-law Edward Kaufmann for their seasoned critiques of the manuscript, to my sister-in-law Davie Kaufmann, and to my parents, Rena and David Aviv, for their everlasting encouragement and love.

Finally, I would like to thank my patients who have been frank about their desire for a holistic approach to their illnesses. I hope that by the writing of this book, I will continue to develop new ways to address their needs.

RESOURCES

Aviv, Jonathan. *The Acid Watcher Diet: A 28-Day Reflux Prevention and Healing Program.* New York: Harmony Books, 2017.

Carrera-Lanestosa, Areli, Yolanda Moguel-Ordonez, and Maira Segura-Campos. "*Stevia rebaudiana* Bertoni: A Natural Alternative for Treating Diseases Associated with Metabolic Syndrome." *Journal of Medicinal Food* 20, no. 10 (October 2017): 933–43. https://doi.org/10.1089/jmf.2016.0171.

Dunbar, Kerry B., Agoston T. Agoston, Robert D. Odze et al. "Association of Acute Gastroesophageal Reflux Disease with Esophageal Histologic Changes." *Journal of the American Medical Association* 315, no. 19 (May 2016): 2104. https://doi.org/10.1001/jama.2016.5657.

Gardner, Elaine. "Alternative Sugars: Agave Nectar." *British Dental Journal* 223 (August 2017): 241. https://doi.org/10.1038/sj.bdj.2017.697.

Gill, Shubhroz, and Satchidananda Panda. "A Smartphone App Reveals Erratic Diurnal Eating Patterns in Humans That Can Be Modulated for Health Benefits." *Cell Metabolism* 22, no. 5 (November 2015): 789–98. https://doi.org/10.1016/j.cmet.2015.09.005.

Kahrilas, Peter J. "Turning the Pathogenesis of Acute Peptic Esophagitis Inside Out." *Journal of the American Medical Association* 315, no. 19 (May 2016): 2077–78. https://doi.org/10.1001/jama.2016.5827.

Lebwohl, Benjamin, Yin Cao, Geng Zong et al. "Long Term Gluten Consumption in Adults Without Celiac Disease and Risk of Coronary Heart Disease: Prospective Cohort Study." *British Medical Journal* 357 (May 2017): j1892. https://doi.org/10.1136/bmj.j1892.

Panda, Satchin. *The Circadian Code: Lose Weight, Supercharge Your Energy, and Transform Your Health from Morning to Midnight.* New York: Rodale Books, 2018.

Schroeder, Bjoern O., George M. H. Birchenough, Marcus Ståhlman et al. "Bifidobacteria or Fiber Protects against Diet-Induced Microbiota-Mediated Colonic Mucus Deterioration." *Cell Host & Microbe* 23, no.1 (January 2018), 27–40.e7. https://doi.org/10.1016/j.chom.2017.11.004.

Wald, Julian P., and Gertrud E. Morlock. "Quantification of Steviol Glycosides in Food Products, *Stevia* Leaves and Formulations by Planar Chromatography, Including Proof of Absence for Steviol and Isosteviol." *Journal of Chromatography A* 1506 (July 2017): 109–19. https://doi.org/10.1016/j.chroma.2017.05.026.

Zou, Jun, Benoit Chassaing, Vishal Singh et al. "Fiber-Mediated Nourishment of Gut Microbiota Protects Against Diet-Induced Obesity by Restoring IL-22-Mediated Colonic Health." *Cell Host & Microbe* 23, no. 1 (January 2018): 41–53.e4. https://doi.org/10.1016/j.chom.2017.11.003.

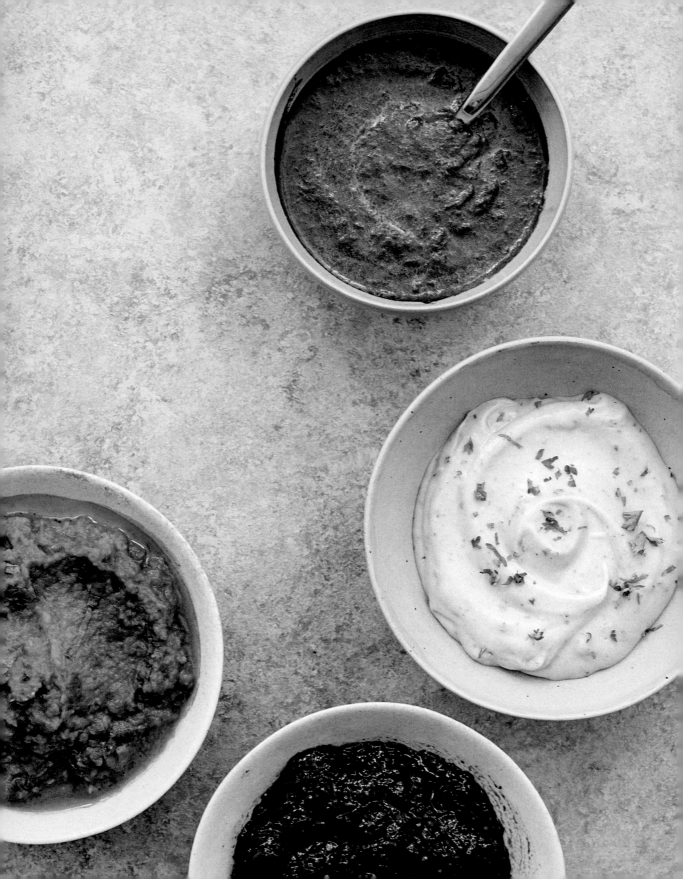

Jonathan E. Aviv MD, FACS

Dr. Aviv is the clinical director and founder of the Voice and Swallowing Center at ENT and Allergy Associates, LLP, in New York City. He is also clinical professor of otolaryngology, Icahn School of Medicine at Mount Sinai. Dr. Aviv is the former director of the Division of Head and Neck Surgery, Department of Otolaryngology–Head and Neck Surgery, College of Physicians and Surgeons, Columbia University.

He is the inventor and developer of the endoscopic air-pulse laryngeal sensory testing technology, known as FEESST. He also pioneered the development of awake, unsedated upper endoscopy, called transnasal esophagoscopy (TNE). Dr. Aviv has authored over sixty scientific papers in peer-reviewed journals and has written two medical textbooks, *Flexible Endoscopic Evaluation of Swallowing with Sensory Testing* (FEESST) and *Atlas of Transnasal Esophagoscopy*. He is the author of the health and wellness book *The Acid Watcher Diet: A 28-Day Reflux Prevention and Healing Program*.

Dr. Aviv is past president of the American Broncho-Esophagological Association and the New York Laryngological Society, and former chairman of the Speech, Voice, and Swallowing Disorders Committee, American Academy of Otolaryngology–Head and Neck Surgery. He is the co-developer of *Project Wellness* with Atlantic Records, featuring the creation of a video on vocal health.

Dr. Aviv has been listed in *New York* magazine's "Best Doctors" in 1998–2013 and 2015, *Best Doctors in America 2004–2018*, *Who's Who in America*, *Who's Who in Medicine and Healthcare*, and *Who's Who in Science and Engineering*.

Dr. Aviv has written blogs for *The Dr. Oz Show* website, Forbes.com, DysphagiaCafe.com, MindBodyGreen.com, and Livestrong.com, and has been featured in articles in the *New York Times* and the *Wall Street Journal*. He has also performed a TNE at the White House for Ronny L. Jackson, MD, physician to the president, and has appeared on *Good Morning America*, *The Dr. Oz Show*, *NBC Nightly News with Lester Holt*, CNN, *Inside Edition*, *Good Day New York*, *The Better Show*, Bloomberg Television, and the Discovery Channel.

Samara Kaufmann Aviv, MA

Samara Kaufmann Aviv graduated cum laude from Colgate University, majoring in psychology and philosophy, and did her graduate studies at New York University in General Psychology, graduating with honors. She subsequently underwent five years of postgraduate training in psychoanalytic psychotherapy, with a special interest in eating disorders and substance abuse. Ms. Kaufmann Aviv is the author of two peer-reviewed studies in the mental health literature.